SUNDAY TIMES BESTSELLING AUTHOR

CASEY WATSON

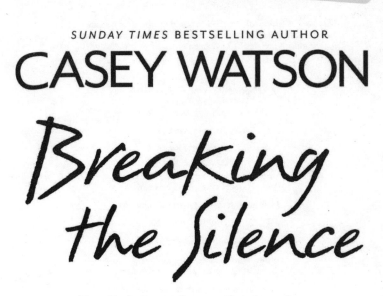

*Breaking
the Silence*

Two little boys, lost and unloved.
One woman determined to make a difference

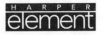

This book is a work of non-fiction based on the author's experiences.
In order to protect privacy, names, identifying characteristics,
dialogue and details have been changed or reconstructed.

HarperElement
An Imprint of HarperCollins*Publishers*
77–85 Fulham Palace Road,
Hammersmith, London W6 8JB

www.harpercollins.co.uk

and *HarperElement* are trademarks of
HarperCollins*Publishers* Ltd

First published by HarperElement 2013

1 3 5 7 9 10 8 6 4 2

© Casey Watson 2013

Casey Watson asserts the moral right to
be identified as the author of this work

A catalogue record of this book is
available from the British Library

ISBN: 978-0-00-747961-0

Printed and bound in Great Britain by
Clays Ltd, St Ives plc

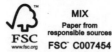

FSC™ is a non-profit international organisation established to promote
the responsible management of the world's forests. Products carrying the
FSC label are independently certified to assure consumers that they come
from forests that are managed to meet the social, economic and
ecological needs of present and future generations,
and other controlled sources.

Find out more about HarperCollins and the environment at
www.harpercollins.co.uk/green

To my wonderful and supportive family

Acknowledgements

I would like to thank all of the team at HarperCollins, the lovely Andrew Lownie, and my friend and mentor, Lynne.

Chapter 1

If you decide to make fostering your career, there's one rule you must be aware of. You should always expect the unexpected. I knew that anyway, of course, because I'd been fostering for a few years now. And before that, I'd worked for years in a similarly testing environment, running a unit for challenging teenagers in a large comprehensive school. And it was one of the aspects I most wanted to impress upon my daughter Riley, now that she and her partner David had decided to take the plunge, and had applied to become fostering-agency respite carers. She was excited, having received her application pack in the post that same morning, and was over at ours telling me all about it.

And how ironic it was that, the very same afternoon, she'd have a chance to see the rule in action for herself. I still smile to myself thinking about it now.

* * *

It was one of those glorious afternoons in mid-June; an ordinary Thursday that had been transformed by the addition of some properly warm sunshine – so much so that we not only managed to spend the afternoon in the garden, but even planned to have tea outside as well. It was also a precious few hours of rest for Riley, David having taken the afternoon off work to take my little grandsons to visit his mum. My husband Mike had just arrived home from work and was upstairs taking a shower, so the pair of us had gone inside to finish preparing a meal of roast chicken and salad, ready to take back outside as soon as he was done.

'I think I've seen enough, with you and Dad's kids, to know what to expect,' Riley laughed, in response to my warning. 'Probably more than enough. More than most have, I'll bet.'

Which was true. We'd only just said goodbye to a gorgeous little girl, Abby, with whom it had been a pretty bumpy ride. Happily, however, she'd left us in the best possible circumstances; she'd been able to be reunited with her mum. Such a happy outcome was a circumstance that was unusual in our line of work, though, because my husband Mike and I didn't do mainstream fostering. We took in kids who had come from particularly difficult backgrounds and as a consequence displayed challenging behaviours. To deal with this, we'd been trained in a specialist behaviour-management programme, with the hope that such behaviours – the sad result of years of psychological damage – could be minimised enough to help them live more settled and fulfilling lives, having hopefully, if not completely banished their demons, found ways to keep them under control.

But being reunited with happy families was mostly a dream for such children, sadly. Ours was very much 'last-chance-saloon' fostering, the expectation being they could at best find permanent foster homes.

'I know,' I said to Riley. 'But seeing it is one thing, and living it is another. You need to go into it with your eyes open. Which is why I think it's such a good idea to do respite fostering first.'

Riley had been keen to press on and apply to be a full-time foster carer, and I still wasn't convinced she wouldn't go ahead. But it was important she lived the reality of it for a bit first – which was why I'd suggested she get some experience doing respite care first. It could take quite a toll on your emotions at times, and with Levi and Jackson still so small, not to mention David working such long hours trying to build his business, I didn't want her drowning under the pressure.

She grinned. 'So you've told me eight million times already, mother – if you hadn't already noticed. Don't *worry*.' She batted her lashes at me. 'See? Eyes very much open. Besides, once I *do* do it, I'll have you around to help me out, won't I?' She chuckled. 'I'll have you on my speed dial. Rent-a-foster gran!'

'Cheeky mare!' I retorted, though I was smiling too. I knew my daughter. And most importantly, I knew *me*. However much I had on my plate with my own foster kids and grand-kids, and my two adult children, I knew full well that what Riley said was absolutely spot on. I'd be in the thick of it. I wouldn't be able to stop myself. They say knowing what you're good at is the secret of a happy life, and I *did* know. Had known the day I had signed on the dotted line with the fostering agency. I loved kids, loved being around them, loved nurturing them and teaching them, loved watching them grow. And once my own two *had* grown, I was the classic empty nester. Though my son Kieron had still been living at home with us till just over a year ago, once he was all grown up I was struck by this huge '*Is that it?*' feeling. How had the time passed so quickly? Oh, yes – I'd had a huge, kid-shaped hole in my life, and at the tender age of only ... erm ... forty-something was, by anyone's yardstick, way too young to take up knitting and bowls. Oh, yes, rent-a-foster gran – bring it on.

And Riley and David would make brilliant foster parents. I knew that too. Although they were still very young, both being only in their twenties, they had recognised there was something of a gap in the market. There were some younger carers but not very many, because, as Riley had pointed out, most people preferred to start their fostering career later in life, once their own children were getting older, or flying the nest. And this, particularly, was why she and David wanted to go into it. They felt that it should be encouraged as a career choice for young couples; with youth on their side, they had just so much energy.

Privately I had absolutely no doubts about them doing it. But that didn't mean *they* shouldn't have doubts; it was a big thing to take on, and not a career anyone should consider lightly.

'So, what about you anyway?' Riley asked me, as we finished off the salad and started piling everything up on to trays to take outside. 'Oi, Dad, keep your hands off that till I say so!' she admonished Mike, who'd now come downstairs, ravenous as usual. He was a big man – six foot three – and his job was physically demanding, and he didn't tend to eat much when he was at work. So it was a full-on job trying to stop him grabbing stuff before I'd even begun to dish up. Right now he was trying to get his hands on a drumstick.

'What, child-wise?' I asked, as we set the plates down on the table.

'Yes. Anything in the pipeline from John?'

John Fulshaw was our fostering-agency link worker. He had been from day one, and we counted him very much as a friend now. But he was still a professional, and he cared about the welfare of his carers. He would generally insist we had a period of rest between each placement so we could recharge both our physical and emotional batteries. 'Not as yet,' I said. 'But then it's only been a couple of weeks since Abby left ...'

'I know,' Riley answered. 'But I always get the impression that he gets them lined up in advance for you. That that's how it works.'

'That's probably how it does work. Why wouldn't it? There's always such demand, sadly. And yes, he probably does,' I agreed.

'He probably tries to, at any rate,' Mike said, chuckling as he sat down. 'I thinks he worries that if he leaves me and Mum too long without one, we'll get too used to the peace and quiet and decide we don't want to do it any more.'

'As if!' Riley chuckled.

'*Exactly*,' Mike said.

'Actually,' I said, sitting down, 'I'll probably call him next week if we don't hear from him before then.' I turned to Riley. 'Dad's got a week's holiday he's got to use up, haven't you, love? So it might be an idea to plan something sooner rather than later. Especially if the weather's looking like carrying on like this ...'

And that – that exact moment – was when the doorbell rang.

My first thought was that it might be Kieron. Our youngest son often showed up unannounced for tea. I sometimes wondered if his sense of smell was superhuman, and that he could catch the scent of a chicken roasting from several miles away. Now 23, he lived with his quite long-term girlfriend, Lauren, at her parents' home. They had a self-contained flat there, which gave them a measure of independence. But not so much independence that I'd be fretting about him all the time. Kieron has Asperger's syndrome, which is a mild form of autism, and means he's a little different from most other people. He is very concrete in his thinking, and particularly averse to surprises. And very trusting – he can see bad in no one.

Kieron, too, was dead set on a career involving children; he'd studied sound production at college, and did regular DJ-ing, but in the past year he'd settled on doing outreach work with youngsters, for a youth centre he'd once been a member of himself. He'd even set up a junior football team for them – he was a talented and committed footballer – so that kids from difficult backgrounds could find a sense of continuity, as well as learning a skill. They'd obviously also learn about teamwork, and get some valuable exercise – one of the best ways to work off their frustrations.

But it wasn't Kieron at the door. I could see that as soon as I entered the hallway. The shape – or rather shapes – though the frosted-glass panel were all wrong.

A neighbour, then, perhaps, I thought as I approached the door. Or some Jehovah's Witnesses … It wouldn't be the postman. Not at this hour.

But it was neither. I opened the door to find John Fulshaw standing on the doorstep, and whose ears, it crossed my mind, must have been burning.

'Hello, Casey,' he said, somewhat sheepishly, as our eyes met. Mine didn't linger, it must be said, because they couldn't fail to be drawn to the small boy standing next to him, who was reluctantly clutching the hand of a third person – a tall red-headed woman, carrying a luminous green holdall, who looked to be in her late twenties and who I would have bet serious money was a social worker. You get a nose for these things, after years working with social services, just as I'm sure other people might say I looked every inch the foster mum. The boy himself – who had almost-black hair, cut long and floppy, in a kind of bowl shape, looked eight or nine, and had an expression I'd seen many times. He looked a highly unwilling part of this little tableau. I swept my eyes over him, assessing him as I did so. Grey school trousers with holey knees, creamy-grey polo – once white – and, tied round his waist, a burgundy school sweatshirt, from which two sorry frayed cuffs hung limply.

'John,' I said, 'I wasn't expecting you! Should I have been? Only you usually call first …'

''I know. I do, and I didn't, and I'm sorry.' To which there was no other than answer than 'Come in'.

So I said it. 'Come on,' I said. 'Though you'll have to excuse the mess. If I'd known you were coming …'

I let the sentence hang and make its point for me. They say a person's house is always cleanest in the ten minutes before visitors are due to arrive, but this is not true in my case. I am something of a clean-freak, as my mother was before me, so it wouldn't be a case of ten minutes before a visitor showed – I would have spent *hours* making everything just so. So I was in something of a flap, casting around for signs of mess and clutter.

John's apologetic expression immediately morphed into a grin. He knew me and my obsessions well. He stepped into the hallway, the small boy and the woman close behind him, and said, 'Trust me, the word "mess" doesn't apply here. Marie – Sorry, forgive me. Casey – Marie. Marie – Casey. You are about to step into the cleanest house *ever*.'

If it was an attempt to mollify me, in the face of this unscheduled visitation, it did the job. You couldn't be cross with John for long. But I was still confused. My mind was whirring, in fact. I looked down at the little boy (though not that far down – I'm five foot nothing) and he looked every bit as dazed and confused as I was. I smiled at him. 'And you are?'

He stuffed his free hand into a trouser pocket, and glanced up at Marie. She gestured that he should go ahead and answer. 'Jenson,' he said finally, eyeing me warily.

'Well, hello, Jenson,' I said. 'I'm Casey. Come on in.'

I raised an arm to usher them all into the kitchen/diner where, from out of the rear window, we could see Mike and Riley tucking into their meal in the warm sunshine – presumably expecting me back, at any moment, from seeing to whoever had been at the door. Which wouldn't be this trio, I thought, smiling to myself.

'So,' I said to John, 'as you can see, we were just having tea. Not that it can't wait,' I added hurriedly, seeing his mortified expression. 'It's only salad.' And it *could* wait. Roast chicken was just as nice cold. I could feel the prickle of excitement I always felt at these times. It really was most odd that he hadn't called me, and I knew there must be a good reason. 'Do you need me to call Mike in?' I asked him.

John nodded. 'Yes, I think so.' He turned to Marie. 'I tell you what, how about you take Jenson out into the garden? That's Riley out there that you can see – Casey's daughter. I'm sure she'd like to meet you, Jenson. Would that be okay?'

9

'Of course,' I said. 'And maybe you'd like a bounce on our trampoline, Jenson.'

The little boy's eyes lit up, and his answering smile completely transformed his grubby face. Is there a child anywhere who doesn't love trampolines?

By now, Riley and Mike had become aware of our little gathering, and as Marie and Jenson stepped outside, and I beckoned Mike in, I caught Riley's eye and grinned at her.

You see? I thought. *Expect the unexpected ...*

Chapter 2

'I'm so sorry, both,' John said, once the three of us were alone in the kitchen, Jenson and Marie having gone outside to join Riley. 'I would have called – of course I would – and I feel dreadful barging in on your family dinner, but this has all been a bit of a mad rush, to be honest.'

'No need to apologise, John,' Mike said. I could tell that, like me, he was just anxious to hear more.

'D'you want a coffee or something?' I added.

John shook his head. 'No, you're fine,' he said. 'I've just had one. Well, half of one, anyway – the other half is still sitting on my desk back at the office.' He grinned wryly. 'I hadn't planned on leaving in such a rush.'

'That sounds ominous,' said Mike. 'What was this – some sort of snatch or something?'

'Sorry,' said John. 'I'm probably making it sound more dramatic than it is. I didn't call *en route* simply because I didn't want to upset Jenson any more than necessary. We've not long picked him up from school – they kindly hung onto him till I could drive down there and meet up with Marie. And bringing him here has all been a bit last minute, to be honest. Otherwise I would have called you before I went to get him, obviously.'

Which wasn't telling me much more about anything. 'So what's happened?' I asked John. 'Why's he been taken into care?'

'Home alone,' he explained. 'You'll be familiar with the film, I imagine?'

We both nodded. 'So we've got a Macaulay Culkin out there, have we?' asked Mike.

'That's about the size of it,' John said. 'Though not quite all alone. There's also a big sister, name of Carley, who's 13. The two of them have been living alone for almost a week now. The mum is apparently on holiday with her boyfriend, somewhere in Spain.'

'Unbelievable,' I spluttered, my eyebrows shooting up. But not for long because, once I thought about it, however shocking it was that a mother could behave in that way, it wasn't *so* unbelievable. Not really. I'd seen too much over the years not to know that first hand. Mike, who was standing with his arms folded, seemed to think the same. He merely shook his head slightly and rolled his eyes.

'I know,' said John. 'Reported by the next-door neighbour, by all accounts, following some sort of house party. She says she knew they were on their own but didn't feel the need to do anything about it. Or didn't want to, at any rate. Marie tells me she didn't really want to get the mum into trouble. But after the party – something of an alcohol-fuelled all-nighter, so Marie tells me – she apparently had a bit of a change of heart. Started to worry that if something actually did go very wrong, then she might get the blame in any case, for not having stepped in and done anything.'

'So where's the daughter – where's Carley? Have you found a place for her?'

John shook his head. 'Not me. She's being placed out of the area. Social services thought it best. If they place her locally they're concerned that she'll simply disappear and go and camp out at a friend's house, in which case they might lose track of her. And also Mum, of course.'

'And what *about* Mum?'

'Marie hasn't been able to make contact with her. And neither have the children for that matter.'

John went on to explain that, according to the daughter's point of view, it was all a big fuss over nothing. They'd been left food, they'd been left money, and they'd both promised to go to school, and as far as she was concerned there was no reason why they should be taken into care. And perhaps, had there been a relative they could have gone to, they wouldn't have been either, except for one crucial thing. The mother's phone was apparently turned off, so the children – like social services – had no way of getting in touch with her. Which, by anyone's standards of acceptable parenting, was simply not on – in fact, it was neglect. And now that they knew about what was happening, social services had a responsibility to step in and act.

'Just incredible,' said Mike, shaking his head again.

'Quite,' agreed John. 'Anyway, so that's where we're at. And obviously why I've fetched up on your doorstep with young Jenson. And the main reason I didn't call first was that I'd originally planned on seeing if I could take him to one of our regular respite carers – in all probability, this is only going to be for a few days or so, after all – but she called back just after we picked him up to say she doesn't want to commit to it any more – had second thoughts as she's got a holiday abroad booked in a week's time, and if it runs over ...' Mike and I exchanged a look. 'Well ... we obviously wouldn't want to send him from pillar to post, would we? And then I thought of you two –'

Who *were* free, of course. In theory at least. 'You don't have a child lined up for the programme right now?' I asked him. In the normal course of events we'd be given a specific child with that in mind. And for a long-ish placement, because the programme took roughly nine months to complete.

'Yes and no,' John said. 'There are a couple of cases going to panel next week, both of which children are potentially suitable to come to you, but as that's likely to take us into the following week – given that they'll need to make a decision and then do an introductory visit and so on ... Well, that was why I had my eureka moment and ended up here. Since this is definitely short term.'

I laughed out loud. 'Oh, John, you are priceless! How many times have we heard *that* before!'

John shuffled on his feet a little, looking like a naughty schoolboy who'd been hauled into a head teacher's office.

Not that it mattered to us whether it was short term or long term. A child who needed a home was a child who needed a home. And if there was a child subsequently who would benefit from completing our specialist programme but as a consequence couldn't do it with us, then so be it. There were other specialist carers. And that was the agency's business. Not ours.

'Fair comment,' John said. 'But, as I say, this time I think it *will* be … Look, I know these cases can be notoriously difficult to second guess – it depends so much on the individual judge on the day – but given the neighbour's comments I see no reason why they won't go straight back to Mum's – rap on the knuckles, some sort of supervision order, and so on. Case closed. And even in the worst-case scenario, which we're not even *thinking* about right now, obviously, well, it would probably be long-term foster care, with a regular mainstream foster family. Which, for a straightforward kiddie like this, shouldn't be too much of an ask. They're okay kids, both of them, according to the neighbour. Though I should tell you,' he added, having obviously had an afterthought, 'that the school is slightly less charmed by our little chap here.' He glanced out of the window, to where Jenson was indeed bouncing on the trampoline. 'Bit of a tendency to truant and also something of a handful, we were told. And that's literally all I can tell you – we were only there a few minutes.'

He looked from one to the other of us. 'So,' he said. 'What do you say? You can obviously say no, because I have no business dumping this on you without warning. And you might have a holiday planned yourselves, of course ...'

Which would have been an easy thing to say, and also true – well, sort of. But I couldn't think of a single reason *not* to step in here, and I knew Mike would feel the same. This was what we did – took in children who needed a loving temporary home. And we could certainly provide that. And one with, by the looks of it, more supervision and more boundaries. You couldn't do a lot in a couple of weeks, admittedly, but you could always do *something*.

'Well?' I began, turning to Mike. 'I'm up for it, if you are, love.' But just as I'd got the words out, we all heard a roar of laughter from the garden. Riley's voice. We all turned to look.

Marie was standing on the patio, Riley seated at the table beside her, both in stitches watching Jenson, who'd evidently become bored of trampolining, execute a perfect Michael Jackson moonwalk across the garden, accurate in every detail, right down to tilting an imaginary trilby hat. Once again, his cheeky grin seemed to light up his whole face, and I got that familiar prickle at the back of my neck.

'One thing,' John cautioned, 'before they come in. We've decided to say nothing to the kids at the moment – you know, about the possible outcomes we discussed. As far as Jenson is concerned, he's just staying with you till his mum gets back from holiday. End of. No point in stressing him any further.'

'Of course,' I said, beckoning the three of them back inside. Poor child. Poor *children*. How could any mother *do* that? I turned back to John. 'And fingers crossed that's exactly how things will turn out.'

A bemused Riley, plus Marie, plus Jenson came in then. 'Yep, this'll do,' he was telling Marie as they crammed through the doorway. 'I'll stay for a bit.' He turned to me. 'Is there owt for tea, though? I'm Hank Marvin.' He grinned at me. (Shyness clearly wasn't an issue here.) 'That means "starving",' he helpfully translated.

I grinned back. 'I think we can rustle something up for you,' I told him. 'Since you're staying.' I was touched by what I reckoned had to be a carefully feigned nonchalance. Deep inside, for all his air of confidence and jocularity, I didn't doubt at least a part of him was anxious and afraid.

'Yeah, well, I'll stop for a bit,' he confirmed.

So that was that then. No paperwork, no pack drill, no lengthy introductions. Just a boy with a green holdall and a promise from Marie to keep us up to speed re any developments. So while Mum basked in the Costa-del-shame-on-you with her boyfriend, it seemed we had a new occupant for our blue room.

Chapter 3

No two cases are the same in our line of business – how could they be? No two children are the same. But you do pick up experience, and a nose for what's what, along the way, and though we'd had to bypass the usual procedure of initial meetings and briefings, what we had here in Jenson seemed pretty straightforward: a little boy who was being brought up by what looked like a fairly neglectful parent. Not the worst parent in the world – and we'd experience of a few in that category – but certainly not one who, on the face of the little we did know, made bringing up her children as much of a priority as some. And that was evident from the minute John and Marie left.

Here was a child clearly used to a fair degree of freedom; used to sorting himself out, while his mum was probably otherwise engaged. As a result, two things weren't terribly high on his agenda: cleanliness and manners.

'I don't want no one goin' in here unless I say so,' he announced, after we'd trooped up to the blue bedroom, and he'd had a chance to inspect it for himself. He waggled his 9-year-old finger at me to press his point home, as well, and I could see that his fingernails were filthy. Had he seen much in the way of soap and water since his mum had taken off? I doubted it. A decent haircut and a shampoo wouldn't go amiss either.

Riley was standing next to me on the landing and I tried not to catch her eye. I knew if I did I'd have trouble keeping a straight face. Ditto Mike, who I could see was struggling mightily.

'Oh, you don't need to worry about that,' he told Jenson. 'We have rules here about people going into other people's bedrooms. Tell you what, how about we go back downstairs, get you a drink and a biscuit, and we sit down and have a chat about how things work here. That a plan?'

Jenson sniffed. 'Yeah, I s'pose,' he said, thrusting his hands in his trouser pockets and yanking them up a little. I could see they had no button.

'And I'd better head back,' said Riley, as we all trooped downstairs again. She checked her watch. 'And get my two to bed. So maybe I'll see you again soon, Jenson,' she said once she'd grabbed her handbag. Jenson sniffed again, noisily, and I made a mental note about nose blowing. 'Nah, I doubt it,' he said. 'I'll be off home soon, I 'spect. Oh an' Mike,' he added, as he followed him into the kitchen. 'Just so you know, I don't do bedtimes.'

* * *

It was nice to let Mike take charge of setting out the house rules. Usually, that was something I'd do, as almost invariably Mike would be at work. He was a warehouse manager – had been for most of his working life – which meant early starts and more Saturday-morning stints than I'd have liked. I also had a hunch that it would be good for Jenson too, as from what little we knew of his home set-up he wasn't used to a great deal of discipline from Mum.

I popped out into the garden with a tray, to clear what was left of tea, and left them to it. I was hoping Mike would be able to get the best out of Jenson now that he'd found himself in the negotiating seat. It was obvious that Jenson thought little of rules and was clearly used to getting his own way. Not so much of a big deal for our family – we'd been fostering a while now, so we were used to this – but something that I mentally added to my list of priorities for this kid.

There was a chill in the air now, and a breeze; we'd clearly had the best of the day already. Then I came in and prepared a plate of biscuits and a glass of squash for Jenson, before stacking the dishes to deal with later and going to join them.

'Right,' Mike was saying. 'So here's what we like to do.' I saw he'd already been to the drawer where we kept copies of our likes and dislikes questionnaire. It was something we'd done from the outset, following on from the training we'd been given; it always helped to settle a child more quickly if you could introduce some continuity by letting them continue doing the activities they liked, watching favourite TV programmes, being given food that they were used to and enjoyed. Mike explained that they'd go through all Jenson's likes and dislikes together, and then quickly run through what was and wasn't allowed in our house.

Jenson looked mildly suspicious as he took a biscuit and began munching on it hungrily. 'Okay,' he said, through his mouthful. 'But I'm not a kid, you know. Like I say, I don't do bedtimes and all that kind of stuff. All you need to do is feed me and wash me clothes if they get mucky. Oh, an' get me up in the morning for school, cos I'm crap at doing that.' He grinned then. 'An' so's me mum. Half the time she forgets to wake me up altogether, and then I get done by the teachers.'

'Oh, dear,' I said. 'Sounds like you could do with an alarm clock.'

'Nah,' he said, ''s okay. It don't matter that much. If they start on me she just goes up and gives them holy hell.'

Once again, I had to fight the urge to meet Mike's eye in case my face cracked.

'Okay,' said Mike. 'And don't worry, we'll certainly do that. And that's the thing, really. That's how things are done at your house, but in our house we play it a little differently. For a start,' he pointed out mildly, 'we don't like using swear words – even "crap" – and we definitely *do* have bedtimes.' He turned to me. 'Casey, what do you reckon is a fair bedtime for a boy of Jenson's age? Let's start with that.'

It took a further half hour of CIA-style negotiating, but we finally had a list of dos and don'ts that Jenson had reluctantly agreed to. We'd set his bedtime as 7.30 p.m. on school nights and 8.30 p.m. at weekends, explained the rules about TV time, and compiled a list of all the foods he liked and disliked, which in the first column included smiley potato faces, pepperoni pizza and chocolate ice cream, and in the second one crab, which he explained he'd been made to eat once and it had made him so ill that he'd been in 'tensish care' for a week.

'They shouldn't call it crab,' he said vehemently. 'They should call it crap!' Then, realising he'd already broken rule one on the list, he looked sheepishly down at his glass of squash.

'Oh, don't worry,' I reassured him. 'We won't give you that. We'd don't eat a lot of crab around here, either.'

'So am I done, then?' he asked, glancing at both of us in turn. 'Can I go and sort my stuff out in my room, then?'

'Go on,' said Mike. 'Fine. I think we're pretty much done here. Off you go.'

Jenson duly trotted off. 'I'll go and put the kettle on,' I said, rising from my chair also, and heading off to the kitchen with the glass and now empty biscuit plate.

When I returned, Mike was grinning to himself. 'What?' I asked him.

'Didn't you hear?' he answered. 'You must need your ears syringing or something. Young Jenson, as he went upstairs, muttering to himself.'

'Saying what?'

'Saying, "This is *well* crap. Just as well it's only a few bloody days." Something along those lines, anyway.'

* * *

But for all our smiles about this uncomplicated-seeming little boy, there was a part of me braced for something darker. He put me very much in mind of Spencer, a boy of around Jenson's age that we'd fostered the previous year. A boy so feral – for all sorts of complicated reasons – that it had been a job keeping him under our roof and safe. For much of his time with us – and he was with us several months – we'd had to keep him almost under house arrest. And when he did get out ... well, suffice to say that we'd been in our present home just six months, and the reason we'd had to move here (which was fine – we loved our new home and neighbourhood) had been directly related to little Spencer. We'd not been asked to go – our landlord was very understanding about our fostering, but after over a decade in our street, our neighbours had actually got a petition together to have us moved, so numerous were the crimes of theft and vandalism and bullying that the cherubic-looking Spencer had carried out. We'd dubbed him a 'one-person walking crime spree' and the description had been accurate. It had been one of the biggest reliefs of our short fostering career that his not inconsiderable family problems had been addressed, and with it, his behaviour as well. He was now back with his mum and, well, so far so good ...

No, I thought, Jenson couldn't possibly be as challenging as Spencer.

* * *

But he was going to be a little challenging – we should expect that as a matter of course. Given the school's warning, the knowledge we already had of his truancy and the fact that, like his sister, he probably thought he should still be at home, we'd be naïve not to see the potential.

And go to school he must. Marie had called us mid-evening, after Jenson had gone to bed, and confirmed what she'd suggested was the case when they'd left us; that they felt it best that Jenson stick to his usual routine, and that meant – seeing as Friday was a school day – going to school. It would be no great hassle, either, because Jenson lived only a couple of miles from where we did, so his primary school was close to our old house. It was also a school I knew well.

Marie also told me the school were fully conversant with Jenson's circumstances, and that they'd be expecting him – well, expecting him-ish, his attendance being generally erratic.

Not while he's with us, I thought, as I went to knock on his door the following morning, just after Mike had had his breakfast and set off for work.

'Morning, sleepyhead!' I said brightly, as I knocked and pushed the door open. 'It's your alarm call – time to get up for school!'

I watched Jenson rub the sleep from his eyes and do a double take at his unfamiliar surroundings, and got the same pang of pity I invariably did faced with a small child, in a strange place, looking bewildered. He shuffled up to a sitting position. His hair was sticking up at all sorts of odd angles, and I wondered whether he'd be amenable to getting it cut.

One thing at a time, Case, I thought to myself, as my eye caught Jenson's open holdall. He'd taken himself off to the bathroom for a wash the night before, and, bar giving him a bath towel – he didn't have one – and showing him how the shower worked, I'd agreed to let him have some autonomy. It was his first night, after all, and I didn't want to smother him. I hadn't heard the shower, but I'd decided not to push it. If he didn't scrub up in the next twenty-four hours, then there might be a bit more personal hygiene supervision, but for now I'd give him the chance to show me he could take care of himself.

He'd obviously pulled out some pyjamas, but it seemed that was all. The bag lay in the corner of the room, sprouting unidentifiable bits of clothing. Unpacked it definitely hadn't been. Taking in the scene, I realised that we were certainly in for a change here. Jenson was a million miles away from our last placement Abigail, a young girl with obsessive compulsive disorder who had been scrupulously clean and tidy. Totally different circumstances, of course, Abigail having been a child carer looking after her severely disabled mother. Jenson, on the other hand, clearly looked after no one – and that obviously included himself.

More alert now, he followed my eye, the notion of 'school' having kicked in. 'I don't wanna go today,' he said decisively, wriggling back down under the covers. 'I just wanna be left alone,' he added theatrically.

'Not up for debate, I'm afraid, love,' I said firmly. 'But it's Friday, at least – last day before the weekend,' I added. 'And then you'll have two whole days off, won't you? So come on. Washed and dressed, please. Or would you like me to help you?'

That had the desired effect. He sat upright again. 'I'm not a bloody kid!' he huffed indignantly. 'All right. I'll get *dressed*, then. I'll be down in a minute, *okay*?'

'Okey dokey,' I said, smiling as I left him to it. 'Oh, but less of the "bloody" if you don't mind. House rules, remember?'

I went back downstairs and set about laying out some breakfast: cereals, milk, sugar, a jug of juice. True to his word, Jenson was down with me just a few minutes later, and though he'd clearly not had time to wash, again I didn't push it. Coaxing him into the shower – and not taking no for an answer – would be on my to-do list for this evening.

Sitting down at my invitation, Jenson, who looked about as crumpled as he would have done if he'd slept in what he was wearing, helped himself to a glass of orange juice. 'Why you got three types of cereal?' he asked me incredulously, as he drank. But before I'd had time to answer, his eyes had moved to the kitchen clock. 'For God's sake!' he spluttered, almost losing his half-mouthful. 'Eight o'clock! Why d'you get me up at *this* time?'

I stifled my grin – from his expression you'd have thought it was 3 a.m. 'School starts at 8.45, love,' I said mildly. 'And you need enough time to wash and eat your breakfast. So chop, chop – you still have to go back up and brush your teeth and hair yet. We can't have you going in looking a state, now, can we?'

Jenson seemed to find the concept of not looking a state a slightly odd one. He poured himself some chocolate crispies and shrugged. 'But,' he said, as if following up on an internal conversation, 'I don't have a toothbrush. I left it at home. And I only brushed them the other day, anyway.'

'Jenson,' I said, 'you are supposed to brush your teeth *every* day. I'm sure you know that. Twice a day, in fact. Morning and evening. So you crack on with your breakfast while I go upstairs and find you a spare one. I'm sure we have one.' And with that, I left him to it and went upstairs.

Once up there, I also had a rummage in Jenson's holdall, in the vain hope of finding some less ropey bits of uniform. But it *was* a vain hope. All the holdall contained was a motley selection of odds and ends: a few pieces of underwear, some mismatched socks, two pairs of limp and grubby jeans, plus a couple of T-shirts that if they *had* seen better days would no longer have any memory of it. I also had a better look at his trainers, which were ancient and filthy. Picking them up, I noticed one had a hole in the sole, too, and I could see where his toes pressed up against the front. I made a note of the size – perhaps my sister Donna would have a slightly bigger pair knocking around that my niece had grown out of.

I put the trainers down again, feeling another familiar pang of compassion. Money didn't buy anyone happiness;

I knew that – but this kind of poverty (or neglect – Mum clearly had funds for foreign holidays, if not new trainers) broke my heart, and I wished I'd had the sense to put his stuff through the washing machine the night before. Or, better still, I should have jumped in the car and slipped off to the twenty-four-hour supermarket in town. I could have had him kitted out handsomely – trainers included – and probably still have had change from forty quid.

I went back downstairs, clutching both a new toothbrush and one of my hairbrushes. 'Here you are, love,' I said, placing both in front of him. 'Try these for size. As in actually *use* them, okay?'

'Will I do now, your majesty?' Jenson asked, with a bow, when he appeared in the doorway minutes later. It looked as though he had simply wet his hands, rather than washed them, and then slicked down each side of his hair. It now formed a ridge across the top of his head like some kind of strange Mohawk. Only very dirty hair could be so precisely arranged.

'That will do just fine, handsome,' I said, smiling at him for at least trying. 'Now come on. After all this hard work, we don't want to be late, do we? So. School stuff? School bag?'

Jenson produced a ballpoint from his pocket. 'Don't need one,' he announced. 'Bags are for geeks.'

And clean clothes, clean hair and clean fingernails as well, I thought, watching with dismay a few minutes later, as Jenson clambered into the back seat of the car, because his knees were almost the same colour as the trousers they poked through. I'd taken grubby children to school before, but this one really took the biscuit. So much so that I was embarrassed to be the person delivering him. *So prepare to become geekified*, I thought as I shut the car door.

Not that I should have worried. Though it felt like a poor reflection on my personal standards, several of the staff knew me well enough, after years of my having kids there (my own as well as foster children), to know these *weren't* my standards. Besides, there were more important things in such situations than a clean uniform, as I was to find out when I popped in, having deposited Jenson with the right teacher, to have a quick catch-up with Andrea Cappleman, the deputy head teacher, just to touch base, really, so we were both up to speed. I didn't know her – she'd not been at the school for very long. But long enough, clearly, to know her charges quite well.

'Don't be fooled,' she warned, ushering me to a seat in front of her desk. 'It's very easy to be taken in by his sweet little "cheeky chappie" persona. He can turn on the charm when he wants to, I know. But there's another side to Jenson. I'm afraid he's something of a bully, and can be extremely disruptive. He also has quite a penchant for taking things that don't belong to him ...'

'I imagine he lacks discipline in his life,' I agreed, carefully, not wanting to jump the gun about a boy I'd known for a scant eighteen hours or so. 'Though, from what I know so far, that doesn't surprise me.'

I didn't want to seem as if I was prying, because it wasn't my place. Not that she had much more to enlighten me with anyway.

'I don't know his mother well,' she said, 'and neither does his class teacher. She didn't come to last term's parents' evening – which would figure, given the fiasco this week – but, as you say, he's definitely a boy who lacks any sort of proper parenting. A boy who'd really benefit from some decent discipline. Boundaries. A few practical lessons in actions and their consequences.'

I nodded. 'Definitely. And that's the plan,' I told her. 'Though I'm afraid we'll probably only be scratching the surface. I imagine he'll be home again by the end of next week.'

'More's the pity,' Andrea Cappleman said, and though she said it with a smile it kind of got to me. She probably didn't mean to – and hers was a hard job, in a big and very mixed-intake city primary school – but I kind of got the feeling Jenson had already been written off as a bit of a pain, which felt sad.

Yes, more's the pity, I thought, as I walked back to my car. Because it *was* a pity. A pity that he'd be leaving us pretty much as quickly as he'd come to us, however much he looked forward to being reunited with his sister and his absent and apparently feckless mum.

Except, as often happens with my musings about future happenings, in Jenson's case it seemed I thought wrong.

Chapter 4

Returning home to find nothing on the answerphone for me, I decided I'd call Marie Bateman.

'What a coincidence you calling now,' she said after she'd greeted me. 'I've literally just put the phone down on Carley Jarvis's carer.'

'And?' I asked.

'And nothing terribly much, I'm afraid,' she told me. 'Still not tracked their mum down, but apparently Carley has confirmed that she is definitely away for a fortnight.'

'So that mean's we've definitely got Jenson till the end of next week then?'

'It would seem so,' Marie agreed. 'Unless Mum shows up any time sooner. But I can't see that happening, can you? And even if she does, she won't be getting the children back, in all likelihood, till she's at least been seen and interviewed.'

'And what about all the children's stuff – clothes and school uniform and toys and so on? Will anyone be going back to the house to collect some more for them?'

'I don't think so,' Marie said. 'I don't think there *was* much more, really. I mean, I could organise someone to go if you want me to, but we did ask Jenson to pack everything he thought he might want to have with him, and from what I saw I'm pretty sure he did.'

So that settled it. Definitely time to break out the plastic. Because I'd made the drive home from school in a very reflective mood. First impressions mattered. Always had, and always would. That was basic human nature. Pride mattered too. As did self-respect. Stuff like that. Perhaps if Jenson could be kitted out to look the part then he'd find it a bit easier to *behave* the part as well. And this wasn't just whimsical thinking on my part. I'd seen it happen on countless occasions in my last job in the comprehensive school. If you treated children with respect, then they tended to behave respectfully. And if a child could feel self-respect, that was a step on the right road.

Besides, I couldn't possibly bear to send *any* child to school in such a tatty uniform. I just couldn't. I said my goodbyes to Marie – her having promised to keep me posted – and left the house again to go and hit the shops.

I shouldn't have really – not without getting John Fulshaw's approval for it anyway. That was the usual protocol, particularly with such a short-term child. You weren't expected to need to run up lots of expenses in such a case.

But equally, I could just throw caution to the wind and hope for the best when I put my monthly receipts in.

I decided to opt for the latter, which didn't take much deciding, because my clean gene prevailed, just as it always did. And I wasn't gone long, either. Within a couple of hours I was back home with my purchases: a new set of school uniform, some trainers and a couple of plain T-shirts, as well as a pack each of much-needed socks and pants. I'd also been a little bit naughty. Struck by Marie's words about just how little he seemed to have, I also went and trawled my usual charity and second-hand shops to see what I could pick up for Jenson there.

Like any mother, I well knew the value of money, and these days, as a foster mother, even more so. So many of the kids we looked after came with hardly anything in the way of possessions, and while we couldn't afford to kit them out with lots of new stuff – we had a budget for such things and we invariably went over it – it was good to be able to give them the sort of clothes and playthings that might have been nothing out of the ordinary for most kids, but was more than these kids had ever dreamed of owning.

And some kids really did come with almost nothing. In one memorable case, a pair of young siblings who'd come from a truly wretched background the previous year had really opened our eyes (eyes that had already been opened) to the extent of the poverty of some children's lives. Ashton and Olivia – who looked a bit like Victorian orphans – had arrived on our doorstep with nothing in the way of possessions between them bar a ripped bin bag, containing just a few scraps of filthy, smelly clothing, and Olivia's grime-encrusted, bald and naked dolly. Polly, she was called, and Olivia loved her very much. Every bit as much as if she'd been the finest doll from Harrods toy department, complete with fine clothes and tumbling golden hair. It had been quite an arresting thing to witness, to say the least.

Some kids, of course, had spent time in the care system, and placements with other foster carers usually meant they had a decent amount of clothing and playthings. But Jenson didn't fall into that category and, given what Marie had said, it seemed clear that he probably didn't have a great deal to his name.

But now he did. Because as well as the clothes I bought him a new football, a schoolbag and, best of all, I had managed to lay hands on a nearly new smart DS games console as well. I felt a bit guilty – I even cringed at the thought of admitting all this unscheduled expenditure to Mike – but something about the way his school had seemed to write him off had got to me, and though he'd so far kept up a fairly solid carapace of nonchalance, how did he *really* feel about the fact that his mum had just swanned off and left him? Pretty sad, I'd have thought. After all, he was only 9.

I don't know if his ears had been burning or not, but Mike phoned me just as I was putting the new clothes into Jenson's chest of drawers. Which meant it was his lunch break. 'How was this morning, then?' he asked me.

'Oh, you know,' I said brightly. 'One or two teething problems when he had to get up for school – no surprises there, then ... ha ha ... but all in all, fine. I did feel bad for him though, love,' I added, as a crafty pre-emptive strike. 'You should have *seen* the state of his school uniform! Those rags he was wearing yesterday? Well, that was the only uniform he had! Can you believe that? Nothing else in there at all! Disgusting, it was, too – God only knows when it last saw some washing powder. You can imagine how happy I was sending him to school in *that* state –'

'So, let me guess,' Mike said, and I was sure I heard at least a hint of a chuckle. At least I hoped so. 'You came straight home from school and then went straight back out again. To the shops, to buy him a new set. Am I right?'

That's the thing with my husband. He knows me too well. And he took it well, too, bless him. And though he wasn't half so understanding when he heard about the DS console, I decided I might as well confess now as leave it till that evening, on the basis that it would at least get his rant (and it *was* a rant) out of the way. After all, it could have been worse. I'd nearly bought him football boots as well.

And I was rewarded, in any case (even if not completely vindicated, given the short time we'd have him with us), by the expression on Jenson's face when we got in from school and we opened the bag. He was thrilled enough on seeing the football, but when he saw the DS the sheer awe on his face was something else. He didn't seem to be able to take it in.

'What, this is for *me*?'

'Yup,' I said.

'What, *just* for me?'

'Just for you, love.'

'What, *only* for me?' It was as if he really couldn't believe it.

'Just for you,' I reassured him. 'A present for you, from us – from me and Mike. Do you like it?'

'Like it?' he almost spluttered. 'It's awesome! It's *epic*!'

'There are a couple of games in the bag, too,' I added. 'I hope they're ones you like. If you've ever played them before, that is …'

'Oh, *yessss*,' he said, pulling the games from the bottom of the bag and inspecting them. 'An' I'm *proper* good at this one – our Carley used to have this one …'

'Oh, she had a DS, did she?' I asked, surprised.

'Yeah, she did. Till she stuck it up on eBay to buy stupid girl stuff, anyway. An' I was never allowed on it. Not 'fically. I could only play on it when she was out an' I could sneak up to her bedroom. Oh, Casey, this is awesome! Can I play on it now?'

'Not quite yet,' I said, grinning. 'I have some other stuff for you as well. There's a new uniform upstairs for you, and a couple of new T-shirts, but before you dash off' – I pulled a box from the counter – 'slip those trainers off and try these on for me, will you?'

Once again, Jenson's face lit up, but then it fell slightly. 'They're a bit clean,' he said doubtfully, as he stamped his way out of his own ratty footwear. He then inspected them, cautiously, as if he were a naturalist coming upon a strange new species of beetle in the rainforest. Approaching carefully, in case they might bite. Then he looked at me with an anxious expression. 'I mean, it's really nice of you, and all, but I don't have to wear them like that for school or owt, do I? I'll get hell if I do, you know. Only geeks wear clean trainers.'

I put the new ones on the floor in front of him and motioned that he should try them, holding the tongues as he wriggled his feet into them. 'They fit?' I asked.

He nodded. 'Seem to, I 'spose, but –'

'Perfect,' I said. 'And don't look so worried, love. By the time we've got through the weekend I'm sure they'll be scuffed up sufficiently for school on Monday ...'

'I hope so,' he said doubtfully. 'Or I'll get picked on like anything.'

Then his lifted his eyes from inspecting his new footwear. 'But I might be home by then anyway, mightn't I?'

Perhaps also due to the wonderful diversionary talents of the DS (particularly for boys of a certain age – clever move, Casey!) Jenson seemed to take it well when I explained that it would probably be another week yet before that happened. And even more so when I explained (again) that since the console was a present it was his to do what he liked with – which meant he could definitely take it home with him when he left.

And Mike too seemed to accept that there was some wisdom in my extravagance – and if it wasn't wisdom, exactly, at least he agreed with the sentiments behind it – that this poor lad obviously wasn't having the best start in life imaginable, and even if we never clapped eyes on him again after this, what was a smallish thing for us – a few quid we couldn't quite afford – it was a gift that might mean something to him. It wasn't that hard to see that, whatever we *didn't* know about his family, what we *did* know was pretty dispiriting.

After an early tea of pizza and smiley-face potatoes ('Well, this is … *interesting*,' Mike commented drily) I asked Jenson if he had any homework to do, and, having been told that they 'never *ever*' got homework on a Friday, let him head back upstairs for another half hour of play.

'After which,' I told him, 'I think you should try out your new football. Isn't that right, Mike?' I asked as we all cleared the table. 'It's a lovely sunny evening, after all.'

They were out in the garden, practising dribbling, when the phone rang.

'Andrea Cappleman,' she said, causing me to glance at my watch. It was gone seven; pretty late for the school to call.

'Oh, this is fairly normal for me on a Friday,' she said. 'I work on the principle that the longer I make myself sit here on a Friday evening, the longer I get to lie in on Saturday and Sunday.'

'That sounds sensible,' I agreed. 'But what's up? Has something happened?' I had a vision of Jenson's mum returning from her holiday and, finding her children gone, kicking down the school door. Or perhaps not. I had a hunch she might not be the type.

'Nothing serious,' she said. 'It's just to keep you informed really. Small incident involving Jenson earlier – got into a bit of a scrap with another boy. I would have called you earlier, but it's been one of those days in school today. And as I said, nothing to worry about; it's just that we like to keep parents – well, in this case, carers, of course – informed. And, of course, given our conversation about discipline this morning …'

'Of course, thank you. I'll ask him about it. What did he do?'

'Just a squabble with another boy – and between you and me, the consensus is that the other boy provoked him. But since Jenson, being Jenson, was about to fly off the handle, and given what's happening at home right now, the teacher thought it best to remove *him* from the lesson, so he wouldn't get himself into any more trouble.'

'I see …'

'Just so you know. Anyway, I'll leave you in peace, then.'

And that was that. No big thing, but it niggled at me even so. Because though I understood the reasoning – what with his mum being AWOL, and his apparent history of disruption, perhaps that was the best approach to take in such a situation. But *was* it? Surely it should have been the other boy who missed his maths lesson? Surely there was a case for that as well?

And it continued to niggle at me when I put Jenson to bed. I felt I *should* mention it, if not least to hear what he had to say about it. I also wondered about whether the school routinely rang his mother to report his apparent regular transgressions.

'It weren't my fault!' he protested, even before I'd said anything. Before I'd got much beyond 'Miss Cappleman called'.

'I know,' I said.

'You do? She said that?'

'Miss Cappleman – we don't use "she" – said the other boy was teasing you.'

'He was! I didn't do nothing! He's just a knobhead. He needs a pasting.'

'Which sort of talk is why your teacher thought it was *you* she'd better remove.'

'But it weren't my fault.'

'But you still have to learn how to control your temper, Jenson. Or it'll always be you that ends up in trouble, whoever it was that started it.'

Jenson looked down into his lap. 'I always end up in trouble anyway,' he grumbled. 'It's *always*' – he lifted his hands suddenly, to form quote marks – '"Jenson's fault".'

Which would have been a pretty unremarkable thing for an average 9-year-old boy to say when he got told off, but for one thing. The flash of something in Jenson's eyes, which caught mine, and seemed to be saying so much more.

I didn't know what, but I also knew my radar for such things worked. There was something more here than the usual boyish 'it-wasn't-me' whining. I might not have him with me for long, but I was intrigued about it. *What?*

Chapter 5

Saturday morning dawned, and that meant football. Football figures large in the Watson family – always has done. And always would do, as well. Our son Kieron loved it, and he was a good player, too. And I could probably count on my fingers the number of Saturdays when Mike hadn't gone to watch him play, while he was growing up. And if there was no match on, then football would be on the agenda anyway – Mike and Kieron would simply watch a game together instead. And since Kieron had moved in with his girlfriend Lauren, the ritual had changed only in that, these days, he would turn up on our doorstep to meet his dad, rather than stumbling downstairs, bleary eyed, from his bed.

At the moment Kieron was playing for his own team. It was the team he'd set up for the teenagers who attended the youth centre he worked for, and who otherwise would probably just be mooching round the streets. Needless to say, we were as proud of him for doing it (given the challenges of his Asperger's) as he was of the bunch of lads he played with.

Lauren didn't usually come with him – she generally spent Saturdays shopping with her mum – but as we had a new kid in, she was keen to come and meet him first; like Kieron, Lauren had a bit of a fondness for our 'waifs and strays'. Though she was doing dance and theatre studies at college, she seemed to have the same interest in working with young people. Her course finished in the summer and she'd already secured a job at a local dance studio, teaching dance to young girls.

'Easy,' said Jenson, meeting Kieron's outstretched fist with his own.

'Easy,' responded Kieron, much to my amusement. I must be slightly out of touch with modern boy-speak, I decided. This was obviously the cool way to meet and greet.

'So, you must be Jenson, I take it?' Kieron continued. 'Well, I'm Kieron and this is Lauren. Which football team do you support?'

'Dunno,' Jenson shot back, as quickly as you like. 'My mum says I should support my legs because they support me.'

'Ah, a joker, eh?' Kieron joshed, though managing to look slightly disapproving with it. 'Well, in this house we love footie, which is where I'm off to soon. Got a match. So I'll see you later on, yeah?'

Jenson's face fell. Not a lot, but it was sufficient for me to spot it. Did he want to be asked along, I wondered?

'I'm good at footie,' he responded. 'An' I got a new football as well. So maybe we can have a kick-about when you get back.'

Kieron glanced at his watch, then back at Jenson's eager face. 'I've got twenty minutes,' he said. 'You want to have a kick-about now instead?'

Jenson's grin answered for him, and I smiled to myself. Here was a boy who could really use a dad or a big-brother figure. I wondered if mum's boyfriend fell into that category. 'I'll get my ball,' he said, turning to go and fetch it. Kieron followed. 'Can you moonwalk?' I heard him ask as they headed off.

'He's a funny little lad, isn't he?' Lauren said, while Mike caught up with some telly and the paper and the boys kicked the ball around the garden. Which was fine – with two energetic grandsons in my life, I kept all my planting aspirations strictly out the front.

'Funny as in ha ha, not peculiar,' she added. We were both sitting by the patio doors, sipping mugs of coffee, watching them. Kieron was peeling off his sweatshirt to make a makeshift 'goalpost' to match the one he'd already made from Jenson's hoodie. Jenson, meanwhile, was trying to scuff up his trainers. I winced, but only slightly. He was a boy of a certain age and disposition. What had to be done had to be done.

'He is,' I agreed. 'Though from what I'm hearing he has something of a temper. I've not seen it myself yet, and perhaps we won't, either. We've probably only got him for ten days or so.'

I filled her in on the circumstances, and watched her grimace, just as we had. 'How incredibly selfish,' she remarked. Then she laughed.

'What?' I said, following her gaze but not understanding what she was laughing about.

'Look what he's doing,' she said, pointing towards Jenson.

'What?' I said again.

'Look. I've been watching him. He's done that twice now. Look – see where Kieron's straightening out his sweatshirt? Look, there. Well, just wait. I bet he'll do it again … there, see?'

I watched as Jenson, while Kieron, busy retrieving the ball, had his back turned, ran across to the tidily folded sweatshirt and kicked it. Not aggressively. Just to muss it up a little bit.

And the next thing, of course, what with Kieron being Kieron, was that he saw it and went back over to fold the sweatshirt up again, because he always needed things to be tidy. Only this was obviously the third time it had happened and he'd cottoned on that it hadn't been accidental.

'Hey, you,' we could just hear him saying. 'Cut that out, okay?'

To which Jenson grinned, and they got on with their game.

Lauren and I exchanged grins of our own. That was classic Kieron behaviour. With his penchant for neatness that sort of thing would really wind him up. But what was inter-

esting was the sharpness of Jenson's mind, in catching on
to it, and I wondered if he'd seen such behaviours before.
Maybe not – maybe he was just a very observant boy. And
also cheeky. I'd have to keep an eye on that.

Once Lauren had gone to meet her mum and the boys had
gone to football I wondered how I should spend my day
with our intriguing new charge. And he *was* intriguing;
every new child that came to us was intriguing. That was
why I loved what I did so much. It was the appeal of the
new and challenging. It was a privilege, opening up your
home to these children, every bit as much as it was a paid
job of work. More privilege than anything, I reckoned,
because it taught you so much, and made you feel connected
to the wider world. I had always remembered something a
school friend's father told me, about why he'd decided to
be a doctor. I'd thought – as I suppose we all do – that it
was about being clever, and using your skill in order to
make people better, but though it was partly that, he
explained, there was something much more instinctive.
He'd first got a glimpse of his fledgling career when he
spent a night shadowing a young doctor in A&E, and the
thing he'd taken away from it was this sense of incredible
excitement – and, of course, privilege – at being present,
and of use, at a time in people's lives when they were at
their most scared and vulnerable. He'd said it made him
feel alive in a way nothing else quite did.

I would never have been so lofty as to say what we did
was quite in that league. I couldn't imagine the stress of

having to save someone who might be dying in front of you, but it had always stayed with me, that, and now I was living my own version. Every child who came to us was vulnerable and scared in some way. And winkling out all the whys and wherefores in order to try and help them was a job I thought I'd never ever tire of.

That said, right now I had an energetic 9-year-old to entertain, and a one-on-one session of gentle probing would be the last thing he wanted. I did toy with the idea of sending him off with Mike and Kieron, but in the end I decided against it. Much as I imagined Jenson would have enjoyed watching a football match, I decided it wasn't fair on Mike to have to take him. He'd had a hard week at work and he looked forward to relaxing with Kieron. Jenson being a largely unknown quantity, and with us being *in loco parentis*, being responsible for him out and about definitely wouldn't be that.

And I was happy enough to entertain him myself anyway, because I was still intrigued by the shadow that had crossed his face the previous evening. We might not have him with us long, but I couldn't switch off my curiosity to find out more about what made him tick.

So once Lauren had gone as well, I told him to turn off his DS (he'd been quietly playing on it since Mike and Kieron had left) and come into the kitchen for a chat.

'So,' I said, 'what do you think you'd like to do today? Go to town for a wander? Go for a walk here? We've got some woods just across the green there, and there'll be baby frogs down there by now ...'

Jenson shrugged. 'Don' mind. Casey? What's up with your Kieron?'

'Pardon?' I said, surprised by the question.

'You know. He just seems, like, a bit weird.'

I laughed despite myself. 'Is that right? No, love. He's not "weird", as you put it. Why d'you ask anyway?' I said, thinking back to my chat with Lauren.

And it seemed Jenson was as well. 'Cos of the way he kept freaking out every time I moved his hoodie.'

'Well, perhaps he's just particular about things being nice and tidy. Nothing wrong with that, Jenson. It's a skill you should try to cultivate, come to that.'

'Yeah, I know,' Jenson answered, having digested what I'd said. 'But it's still a *bit* weird …'

'Which is presumably why you kept doing it then, is it?'

Jenson looked at me sharply. He obviously hadn't clicked that we'd seen what he'd been up to. 'To wind him up?' I asked mildly.

'Anyway,' he said, rapidly changing the subject, 'shall we go down the woods, then? I *hate* goin' round shops. Goin' round shops is for girls.'

I'll bet you hate it, I thought. And not just because it might be a 'girl' thing. With no money to buy stuff, why would he want to go shopping? And as a boy with just a sister and a mum to grow up with, my hunch was that he'd spent more time than he wanted doing just that.

'And we'll take a picnic, I think,' I decided, having checked the sky for rain clouds. There were none. 'You like picnics?'

'I love picnics,' Jenson said delightedly. Which delighted me as well. 'An' we can maybe catch some frogs?'

I smiled. 'We'll see. But no crabs.'

'*Definitely* no crabs,' he agreed.

Biology not being my strong point, I wasn't sure if we could expect to see any crabs anyway – they lived on the coast, in the main, didn't they? Anyway, we didn't see any, edible or not. And we didn't catch any frogs, either, except to hold in our hands briefly, as I managed to persuade Jenson that, much as I understood his wish to keep one, I didn't have a frog aquarium knocking around at present, and that he'd be going home soon, in any case, so there wouldn't be a lot of point.

By the time we'd finished our pond dipping and picnic, his trainers were good and filthy, and, though I knew this was the outcome he'd hoped for on this occasion, I decided I should stock up on wellies for my future foster children, as the proximity to the wood and stream meant we'd need them. It was such a wonderful thing to have within walking distance of the house, and I envisaged spending lots of happy hours there.

And the day passed as calmly as did any other Saturday; the evening too. Lauren returned, and she and Kieron stayed for a take-away, and once they headed off, and Jenson trotted up to bed with his DS, I reflected that this might be what mainstream fostering might be like. Relaxed, non-confrontational, nice.

I said as much to Mike. 'It would just be so different, wouldn't it? Like having a succession of chirpy, pint-sized lodgers in the house. And you could easily have more than one, couldn't you? I can so see that.'

'Love,' Mike said, 'have you been watching that *Sound of Music* DVD again?' he laughed. 'Pint-sized lodgers! What are you like?'

I hit him with my copy of the *Radio Times*. 'Cheeky so-and-so!'

'Come on, Case,' he persisted. 'That's so not your thing. I know you. You've never been any different. You get that glint in your eye and you're off –'

'What d'you mean, "off"?'

'Off on one of your save-the-world projects. Love, if you haven't got a problem kid to straighten out, you're bored.'

And he was right, of course. When you're young you don't always know what job's best going to suit you. But when I hit my thirties and got the role running the 'unit' at the comprehensive, it was like a light had pinged on in my brain. I'd come home from work in the evenings, and poor Mike wouldn't get a word in. I would always be 'You won't believe what's happened with this kid', or 'Her mother did this to her – God, I'm horrified', or 'And this one kid said to the other … and then this other one did so and so …' Yes, on reflection, perhaps Mike was right.

Still, I thought, sometimes a rest was a bonus, and we'd definitely had that; so far it had been a perfectly pleasant weekend.

Sunday continued in similar fashion. This time Riley and David and the little ones had come over, and we enjoyed a big family mid-afternoon roast – with Mike's special gravy, of course – all of which seemed to delight Jenson.

'I like little 'uns,' he said, in response to my comment about how patient he had been with Levi and Jackson.

Once the meal was over, we'd all assembled back in the living room, where he'd spent ages trying to teach Levi how to moonwalk.

'I can tell you do,' I said. 'You're a natural, you are, Jenson. You'd make a brilliant teacher, you know. Because you're patient. And that's a very important thing to be.'

He swelled with pride. Literally. Puffed out his chest and lifted his chin up. Then he seemed to think for a minute, watching me getting out one of my cigarettes. My first of the day. A real treat. 'You know,' he said, gesturing towards it. 'If you ever want me to keep an eye on them for you – you know, while you go an' smoke that ...'

I laughed. What a quaint and random thing to say, I thought. 'No need,' I told him. 'It's not a real cigarette, see?'

I handed it to him. It was a plastic one – a nicotine inhalator. The only kind I 'smoked', since making the momentous decision to absolutely, definitely, completely give up smoking. And I'd been doing well so far. Fingers crossed I could keep it up.

Jenson inspected it for a moment before handing it back to me. 'That's *weird*,' he said.

'Yes, but weird in a good way. Weird in a brilliant way. And listen, don't you ever think taking up smoking's big and clever. Once you start, it's very, very, *very* hard to stop.

Anyway,' I said, 'time for a bath for you, I think. School in the morning –'

His face fell. 'Do I have to?'

'Yes, Jenson, you definitely *have* to.' I popped my 'cigarette' onto the coffee table. 'Because those are the rules in this house. And I'll come up with you, if you like. Pop your new pyjamas in the airing cupboard so they're nice and snug and warm to put on afterwards.'

'Aww, okayyy,' he said. And there was something about the smiley way he said it that told me he quite liked having rules after all. Especially when they came with warm pyjamas.

Sorting the pyjamas out, while Jenson took himself off reluctantly to the bathroom, I wondered again about that. Had he ever had his jim-jams warmed before? And what was his mother doing right now – right this minute? Having her first cocktail of the evening? Still lying on a beach somewhere? Canoodling with the boyfriend? But my reverie was interrupted by the house phone.

'Can you grab that, love?' I called down to Mike, knowing it would probably be my mum. She and my dad were pretty much the only ones who ever called the house phone. Among friends and family, at any rate. And who else would be calling on a Sunday evening?

Silly me. Naïve me, not to expect the unexpected. Because it wasn't Mum, wanting to hear all about our new temporary house guest. It was John. With some stuff to tell *us*.

'Here,' said Mike, passing me the phone as soon as I'd come down. 'You might just as well get the latest as me.'

I took the phone, smiling to myself – Mike was in the middle of watching something on telly. Which he wouldn't want to miss. 'John,' I said. 'To what do we owe the pleasure?'

'Good,' he said. 'You're clearly in a good mood. Which is good.'

'I know I say it all the time, John, but that sounds ominous,' I answered.

'Only slightly,' he reassured me. 'It's really just an update. It seems young Carley has been pulling the wool over all our eyes.'

'Oh,' I said. 'In what way?'

'As in she's tried to throw us off the scent, the little minx. Seems nothing in this whole business is as it seems.'

'Go on,' I said, intrigued.

'Well, it's all down to the quick-wittedness of the other foster family, really. Call it what you like – invasion of privacy, snooping, an outrageous bit of shameless spying – but when Carley left the family laptop unattended yesterday they saw an opportunity to do a bit of sleuthing.'

I chose to call it quick thinking. Good on them ... 'And?' I asked.

'It was a gift; she'd dashed upstairs to answer her mobile, which was in her bedroom ...'

'You mean she didn't have it duck-taped to her person?' I asked incredulously. 'What kind of 13-year-old *is* she?'

John laughed. 'Well, that was the gift. Her phone was on charge, so on this occasion, no, she didn't. And the other gift was that she was logged into her Facebook page.'

'A gift indeed!'

'Exactly. So foster mum – I wish she was local; she sounds like my kind of woman – had a quick click and established she and Mum had been messaging each other ...'

'And?'

'And the most important one, for our purposes, anyway, was the one which said "Be back on Sunday – with my Malaga tan. Landing in Manchester about 7."'

'What, as in today? As in tonight? As in she's – I checked the time – only just landed?'

'Indeed she has. This message was sent only the day after we picked the kids up.'

I thought for a moment. 'But why would she tell you she was coming home next week, then?' I asked John. 'It makes no sense.'

'It didn't to us, either,' John agreed. 'But then Marie made the point that she probably didn't know quite what *to* do. Perhaps she panicked. Or perhaps the opposite. Perhaps she had a really cool head on her shoulders, and decided the best plan was to intercept her mother before social services could speak to her. Which does make sense. It would give her a chance to give her the lowdown, and time for them to concoct some sort of story. Or perhaps another explanation is that there's been contact between them since they were taken into care and Mum has curtailed her fortnight's break as a consequence. Anyway,' he added, 'who are we to second guess the workings of a teenage girl's mind? We'll find out soon enough, though. Because Marie'll be there to meet her.' He paused. 'And, of course, arrest her.'

The protocol in such situations is straightforward. Assuming everything went to plan, there would be a police officer at the airport and, while Jenson was putting on his pyjamas upstairs, his mum Karen would be in the process of being arrested – in all probability for wilful neglect. She'd then be released on bail – also normal in these circumstances – and ordered to appear in court at the next available hearing, which in all likelihood would take place the next day. She'd also be informed that her children had been taken into care, though not where they were. She'd also be told not to contact them. Instead she'd be granted supervised contact only – again, within the next day or two.

'Okay,' I said. 'So what'll be the situation now with Jenson?'

John pondered, and I wondered if I needed to say anything to him at all, really. As far as Jenson knew his mum wouldn't be home till the following weekend, after all. Was there anything to be gained from muddying this issue tonight? I didn't think so. Best to wait and see how things panned out. I said as much.

'Actually, I think yes,' John said. 'On balance, I think you should tell him. Best to be straight with him. Just explain that she's come home a bit early and that he'll be able to see her in a day or two.'

I agreed I would. But if his mum's early return was to prove a surprise to Jenson, it was as nothing compared to the surprise *I* had coming.

Chapter 6

Though John's news had come as something of a surprise to me and Mike, it seemed that wasn't the case for every member of the household that evening.

Having relayed the gist of things to Mike (having first given him an opportunity to record what was left of his programme), I asked him to get Jenson out of the bath and ready for bed, while I got some crumpets and a hot drink organised downstairs and decided how to best broach the subject.

Jenson had seemed reasonably accepting of things all weekend – at least, if his mood had been anything to go by, that would have seemed to be the case. He'd asked us barely anything about what had happened and what might be happening to him, and had at no point seemed more than very mildly upset. I'd put it down partly to bravado and partly down to circumstance. If this holiday was typical of the way his mum ran her family, then perhaps her absences were something he was used to. And if being whisked away to stay with strangers was something he wasn't used to, perhaps the compensating factors of free toys and some attention were sufficient for him to maintain his equilibrium.

I'd keep it simple, I decided, as I heard him thunder, in typical 9-year-old fashion, down the stairs, presumably following Mike's directive. Just give him the facts and keep it light, I decided. Tell him he'll be seeing his mum soon.

'Sit yourself down at the table,' I told him, as I popped two crumpets in the toaster. Crumpets were a big thing in our house; our first foster child, Justin, had always loved them, and the habit of getting them in for our foster kids had stuck. 'I just need to have a little word with you,' I added. 'That's all.'

Jenson sat down at the kitchen table and looked expect-ant and slightly nervous. 'Have I done something wrong?' he asked.

I shook my head. 'No, not at all. No, it's nothing for you to worry about.'

'Mmm,' said Mike, joining us at that moment, 'they smell good, love. I hope you've got enough there for me as well.'

'Well, if you're *very* good, I might have,' I said, pulling out the first two. I turned to Jenson as I buttered them. 'It's just that we've had a phone call from John, love. You remember John? The man who brought you here?' I passed him the crumpets and popped two more in the toaster.

'Yeah, I do,' Jenson said, taking the plate. 'What did he want?'

'Well, I don't know if you knew,' I said, watching for his reaction, 'but your mum got back from holiday tonight …'

Jenson's expression changed immediately – and to a configuration I knew well, because I'd been around kids for a long time. Ah, I thought. *Ah*. 'Did you know anything about that?' I asked him mildly.

He was taking a bite from one of the crumpets, and shook his head as he chewed it.

'You didn't know?' Mike asked.

'No,' Jenson tried to say from behind his mouthful. He swallowed. 'No,' he said again.

Which denial should have come out as a 'Yes'. I was sure of it. Because a blush was creeping steadily across his cheeks now.

'Jenson,' I said, 'remember what the rules are in this house. We tell the truth. *All* the time.' I kept my gaze on him.

'I didn't –' he began.

'Jenson,' Mike said. 'The truth, now, kiddo.'

This seemed to work. His expression changed again, this time to one of resignation. 'I didn't know she was goin' to be back, *honest*, I didn't! Just that I had to go meet our Carley. That's all she told me.'

'Go and meet her?' I asked him, confused. 'Meet her when? Meet her where?'

'Last break tomorrow,' he said. 'She was goin' to come an' fetch me,' he admitted.

'Fetch you from school?' Mike asked.

'No, not school. I was s'posed go an' meet her round the corner.'

'But *from* school? In school time, you say?'

Jenson nodded.

I pulled the second pair of crumpets from the toaster. Mike was ready with his plate, even before I started buttering them. 'And then what?' he asked Jenson, still keeping things conversational and non-confrontational.

Jenson shrugged. 'An' then … I dunno …'

'You were going to meet up with Mum?'

He shrugged again. 'Dunno.'

'When did you arrange this?' I asked him.

He eyed the rest of his crumpet, seeming unsure whether to finish it. 'Sweetheart, eat it up,' I said. 'It'll get cold. Like I say, you're really not in trouble. We just need to know what's been going on, that's all.'

Jenson chewed as instructed while I passed Mike his two. 'Was it last week?' I said. 'Before Marie – you remember the lady from social services – came?'

Jenson nodded. So it seemed they'd already planned their reunion! No wonder he'd appeared so relaxed about everything. This stay was going to be nothing more than a weekend mini-break for him! 'But what were you planning to do with Carley tomorrow, Jenson?'

'Go home,' came the immediate response. 'Go home with Mum.'

I sat down now, with a big mug of strong, steaming coffee. So he *did* know his mum was coming back. Had all along, it seemed. 'But sweetheart, I'm afraid it doesn't work like that,' I said gently. 'Because your neighbour –'

'She's just a nosy old bat,' Jenson said with feeling.

'Kiddo, I know it's hard,' Mike said, patting Jenson's forearm. 'But it's not that simple, I'm afraid. Because your neighbour called social services – and not because she was being nosy – because she was worried about the both of you – well, that means they have to have a little chat with Mum first. You can't just go home as if nothing has happened …'

'But nothing *has* happened!' protested Jenson. 'I haven't done anything wrong. I've been a good boy since I been here with you two, haven't I?'

And wasn't that just the nub of it? This poor kid thought it was all about whether he'd done anything wrong. Not his mum – not the one who bore the guilt in all this. No, he was just worried that he might not be able to go home if we gave a poor account of his behaviour with us. Which was sad. Just so sad.

'Yes, you have,' Mike reassured him. 'Very good. But it's not about that, Jenson. They have to chat to your mum to make sure she … well, that she understands how to look after you properly. They need to be sure she's not going to go on holiday and leave you and your sister on your own again. Which is why –'

'So you're telling me I can't go home?' I could see Jenson's chin start to wobble, as the reality of the situation was beginning to sink in. Bless him, he was *9*. He shouldn't have to deal with all this.

'Not that you can't,' I tried to reassure him. 'Just not tomorrow, that's all. But you'll be able to see Mum – they're going to call us in the morning and you'll probably at least be able to see her on Tuesday, and then –'

'But they can't do that!' Jenson interrupted, scraping his chair back. His eyes were swimming and he was struggling not to cry. 'They can't tell my mum what to do, and neither can you!'

'Jenson, son, calm down –' began Mike.

'You *can't*!' Jenson shouted now. 'And neither can some shitty judge! I'm off home tomorrow and you can't stop me!'

'Jenson,' I said, rising as well, 'calm down, love. You'll be seeing Mum very soon. It's like Mike said …'

'Fuck you!' he shouted, the tears flowing down his face now. 'Just you keep out of our business, okay? I'm off home, and if you don' let me, my mum'll come round here and she'll kick your door in. She will, you know!' he added. 'Don't think she won't cos she will! She'll kick your fucking door in!' At which point he rushed out and thundered back up the stairs. We heard the bedroom door slam moments later. Mike picked up his uneaten crumpet and inspected it.

'Well, that went well, didn't it?' he remarked drily.

I woke with the dawn the next morning, and my first anxious thought was that Jenson might have absconded while I slept. When you've previously fostered a child – as we had – with a habit of absconding, the anxiety about a child doing so really never goes away. But when I crossed the landing and peeped in he was still in there, curled up and sleeping soundly, so I quietly pulled the door closed and headed downstairs to brew some coffee.

Not that it wasn't still an issue. I didn't doubt the only reason Jenson was still with us was that he was still committed to plan A – to meet up with Carley as they'd arranged. So the first thing I'd need to do once I'd dropped him at the school gates would be to follow him in – at a suitably discreet distance – and go and speak to Andrea Cappleman.

We'd left Jenson to calm down a bit the previous evening before going up to him, and when we had finally done so he'd already been fast asleep. Which meant that by the time I went to wake him, an hour and a half or so later, he would have slept for a solid twelve hours.

But it seemed he hadn't. Not quite. Because when I went in to him he was already awake, washed and dressed – even if it was in his tatty old uniform. But he obviously *had* washed, which was gratifying to note – there were tendrils of damp hair clinging to the back of his neck. Not that I could see a great deal of him. Though he must have heard me knock, he didn't turn around to greet me. He just remained standing with his back to me, staring (presumably moodily) out of his bedroom window into the street.

'How you doing, sweetheart?' I asked him.

He ignored me.

'Love, I know you're upset,' I said. 'Of *course* you are. But we'll get all this sorted out, I promise.' I was aware that I had to choose my words very carefully – no promises about when he'd be back home with Mum because I had no idea when that might happen. Or even *if*, in fact. The grim possibility was always there, sitting on my shoulder. I knew nothing of this family or what had happened before with them. And nor did social services. But now they did know, there was no telling what they might uncover. It didn't look likely (Jenson didn't bear the hallmarks of an abused child) but the possibility was there, even so.

But that was all it was. A slim possibility. I must keep positive, and so must he. 'In fact, the first thing I'm going to do,' I said 'just as soon as I've dropped you off at school, is going to be to call Marie and find out when's the absolute soonest you can see your mum, okay? And as I say, if not today, then –'

'But *will* you?' he asked me, finally turning around now. His face was pinched and wary, and I had to keep remembering I was a stranger to him. 'Will you *really*?'

He sounded so forlorn and world weary about it, as if he'd been let down by adults all his life. Which perhaps he had. How would I know? I knew almost nothing about him either.

'Of *course* I will,' I said, making a cross on my chest with my finger. 'Cross my heart and hope to die, see?' This seemed to help convince him. 'But, Jenson, love, could you please put your new school stuff on for me? You'd look so much better if –'

'Do I *have* to?' He sighed. 'It's all so geeky, that stuff. An' it's scratchy, too. I feel so much more comfortable in me own stuff.'

Which was a plea that I did have some sympathy with, much preferring my usual combo of loose top and leggings to anything starchy or formal or buttoned up. But I persisted anyway, because uniform was one of life's realities. And growing up was all about accepting life's realities, which was why parenting was all about introducing them. 'It'll soften up,' I promised. 'Just as soon as you start wearing it. And besides,' I added, having had a moment of inspiration, 'just think how lovely it will be to look so smart for your mum. She'll be well proud of you.'

He weighed this up and eventually seemed to accept it. 'Okay,' he said, grudgingly. Then his eyes widened slightly. 'An' what about my DS, as well? I could take it to school, so's I'd have it with me, then I can show it her –'

I shook my head. 'No, you can't, love. You know the rules.'

'But not to get out in class or anything,' he persisted. 'Just to keep in my bag till I see Mum, an' that.'

I shook my head a second time. 'Love, those sorts of things aren't allowed in school, are they? You know that. Tell you what, though – how about I pop it in *my* bag so that when I come and pick you up, if it *does* turn out we can take you to see Mum this afternoon, then we'll have it ready, yes? That a plan?'

That was a plan, he agreed.

And when he came downstairs to eat his breakfast, he seemed quite pleased with his new look. I could tell by his little swagger as he walked into the kitchen, and by the way he carefully arranged his hair in the mirror first, unaware that I could see him through the open door.

'You look like the bee's knees!' I observed as he appeared, ready for inspection. I could tell he was slightly self-conscious now, bless him. 'No I don't,' he said. 'I probly look more like a spice boy. That's what Gary, me mum's boyfriend, would call me in all this kit. What's a spice boy, anyway, Casey? Do *you* know what it means?'

I almost burst out laughing. 'I have absolutely no idea,' I laughed. 'But it sounds just fine to me.'

Though, just to be on the safe side, I made a mental note to ask Kieron. You never knew with boy-speak, after all.

Spice boy or otherwise, Jenson had gone into school happily enough, and promised me faithfully that he wouldn't do anything silly. I didn't know if I could trust him on that point, obviously, and, given the circumstances, I perhaps shouldn't, but, having seen the deputy head and filled her in I at least felt confident she'd make the necessary staff aware of the situation so that they were alert to the possibility that he might.

That done, I decided I needed a quick grandson-fix, so before heading home to tackle the housework I descended on Riley. And via the sweet shop, with an armful of goodies that I knew my daughter wouldn't approve of, but that my grandchildren definitely would.

Well, Jackson would, anyway – Levi would be in nursery all morning, and would have to wait for his treats till a bit later. In the meantime it was nice to linger over coffee, have a natter, and allow myself the luxury of a plastic cigarette, before meandering home to start my traditional Monday cleaning routine.

But by the time I left Riley's I still hadn't heard from Marie, and, feeling guilty that I'd reneged on my promise to call her, I phone her office as soon as I got home again. That it went to voicemail was no surprise – perhaps she was even at the hearing as I was ringing, but it also made me think, when I heard the house phone ringing a couple of hours later, that it would be her, returning my call.

I was upstairs at the time, mopping the bomb-site of a bathroom – not to mention marvelling at how one small (and clearly not terribly fastidious) boy could make such an unholy amount of mess in a confined space. So, having peeled off my Marigolds and parked my soggy mop, it had rung for several seconds before I reached it.

'Hello?' I said, having made a dive for the receiver. 'Marie?'

A throat was cleared, and then I heard a female voice I recognised. 'Er, no,' it said. 'It's Andrea Cappleman from school. Sorry to bother you. And please don't panic – it's just that we have something of a situation, I'm afraid.'

'A situation?' I parroted back at her. 'What sort of situation? What's he done?'

She cleared her throat again, and it was that which made me twig. Perhaps he hadn't done anything. Perhaps it was less 'What's he done?' and more 'Where's he's gone?' And it turned out that I was spot on. 'I'm afraid he seems to have left the premises,' she admitted. 'About half an hour ago.

At least, we think so. He asked the teacher if he could go to the toilet, and, well, it seems –' the throat was cleared again – 'that he never returned. I'm so sorry.'

Sorry? I thought incredulously. Such ineptitude! How stupid did you have to be to fall for that old 'going to the toilet' lark? And what was with the 'don't panic' directive, in that case? He was 9 and he'd absconded. I duly panicked.

'But surely they *knew* that this might happen –' I began, a touch snappily.

But Andrea Cappleman was quick to interrupt me. 'Jenson's teacher *did* know,' she said firmly, and only very slightly apologetically. 'But she'd been called to an incident in the hall – it had to be her that attended it; she's our first-aider – and another teacher had stepped in to keep an eye on her class. We're a busy school, and I'm afraid Jenson isn't the *only* pupil we have to think ab—'

Now it was my turn to interrupt. I'd obviously jumped in a bit hastily. And having done so, I now regretted it. And rightly so. I'd spent plenty enough years on her side of the fence. 'No, no,' I said. 'Of course he's not. I completely understand. I'll get onto his social worker right away. I imagine he'll have gone to meet his sister, as planned. Thanks so much for letting me know.'

I hung up and felt guilty for having been so cross. It wasn't her fault. Or the teacher's. Or anyone's really. These things happened. I should have realised that if Jenson was that determined to meet his sister, then it was odds on he would have found a way to do it, incident or no incident. And of course he *was* that determined. He wanted to see his mum. And there was nothing Mike and I said – two complete strangers who he'd been dumped with for a few days, let's face it – that would be able to do anything to alter that fact.

So, cross as I was that he hadn't done as he was told, I did have some sympathy for him, poor lad. He was just doing what he thought he had to do. What his sister – and mum? – had told him. And something else struck me: no wonder he was so keen to take the DS to school with him. He was working on the basis that, if he didn't, it would be the last he'd ever see of it.

I dug out my mobile and dialled Marie again. Hopefully she'd have forestalled Carley – even intercepted the pair of them. And hopefully the court hearing had happened and gone well. And hopefully – even if this was a *big* ask, in hope terms – the children's mother would have given a decent enough account of herself that she'd be able to have the pair of them back.

Though as the number rang, I couldn't help thinking about all those hopefullys. What was that phrase they used? When people kept on getting divorced and then remarried? The triumph of hope over experience, that was it.

I had lots of the latter, so perhaps, under the circumstances, just a little bit too much of the first.

Chapter 7

I managed to get hold of Marie straight away.

'I'm sorry I've not called you yet,' she apologised immediately. 'I know John's put you in the picture – at least, I assume he has – has he?'

'Yes, yes,' I answered. 'It's –'

'It's just that the hearing was scheduled for p.m. rather than a.m., so I don't have any news yet, and –'

Now it was my turn to interrupt. 'I do,' I said, getting straight to the point. This was no time for chit-chat. 'Jenson's absconded from school.'

Marie groaned. 'Now, why doesn't that surprise me?'

'Exactly,' I said. 'So I'm assuming he's gone to do what he admitted was the plan: meet up with his sister and head home to see Mum.'

'And of course, she might already be on her way home from the hearing by now, too. I need to get round there. We need to get round there ...'

'Absolutely. So if you can let me have the address?'

Marie reeled it off for me. I didn't need to write it down. It was local, and I knew it. I just made a mental note of the house number.

'Okay,' I said, pulling off my apron. 'Thanks. I'll get going, then. Let's just hope it doesn't become unpleasant. And what should I say to her if I get there before you?'

'Which you probably will, because I'm bound to get stuck in traffic. Just keep it light. Tell her who you are and that you were worried about him running off. Tell her you don't know any more than that. I think that's the best way.'

This was actually the truth, I thought, as I jumped in my car and fired the engine. And Marie didn't know much more because she hadn't yet been told the outcome of the hearing. It was perfectly possible the judge had decided to let the children go home. Either way, Marie had assured me that she'd find out before she got there.

Jenson's estate was a big sprawling one, built in the fifties or sixties; certainly at a time before everyone had cars. Every road I drove down had a ribbon of them on either side, all of them listing a little, looking like rows of sleeping animals, half up on the pavement, half in the kerb, leaving just a sliver of road to squeeze my car through. I had to park way past the house, which was showing no signs of life – but which perhaps wouldn't, given this was a sunny early summer afternoon. I hurried back and headed up the front path – there was a gate, but it too was listing – but my knocks on the blue-painted front door produced nothing but an empty echo, which reverberated down the equally empty hallway I could see through the heavily frosted glass.

Not that this meant anything. He wasn't going to answer the door, was he? If he was smart, which I thought he was, he would have been keeping an eye out. He would want to see who was out there before risking revealing himself. And if he didn't like what he saw then he would simply lay low – with or without his older sister.

There was little I could do except wait for Marie to arrive. And then, presumably, for Karen to show up. I stepped back from the door and scanned the street. Jenson could be anywhere. He'd probably have dozens of friends he could go to. It was a huge estate, and one I knew well from my days as a school behaviour manager. I used to visit families here regularly, as part of my job involved visiting troubled kids in their home settings and talking to their families about how they could help their kids better. I'd sit and discuss strategies, talk about boundaries and discipline, then I'd help them create reward charts – I'd always come armed with stars and stickers – to help them try and curb their teenagers' less delightful behaviours.

It seemed a long time ago, now, and in some ways it was. I'd been fostering for almost half a decade now; some *very* intense years.

I was just reflecting on how much my life had changed since I answered that fostering agency ad when I became aware of a 'psst!' sound close to me. I turned to see a woman on the doorstep of the neighbouring semi, silently beckoning that I should step a little closer.

She wore one of those old-fashioned wrap-around aprons that look like dresses, and drew a finger to her lip as I approached. 'Are you one of the social workers?' she wanted to know.

I shook my head, and keeping my voice low to match hers I explained that, no, I was Jenson's foster carer.

'My name's Casey,' I added. 'Do you know something about his whereabouts?'

She cocked her head back. 'The lad's in my garden,' she told me, 'waiting for his mum to get home. Playing with my dog. He loves my Sabre, he does. I expect he's missed him.'

She looked to be in her sixties, and had that bustling, sleeves-up, no-nonsense air of a woman used to looking after herself. I imagined Sabre as a hulking great Alsatian, and her motto to be 'I speak as I find'.

'Come in to the front room,' she commanded, gesturing with her hand as she led the way into her hall. The house smelt of lavender polish, with an undercurrent of onions. She'd obviously been cooking. Something wholesome, I didn't doubt. 'So's he won't see you,' she elaborated. 'Though what you're going to do with him, I don't know. He's bound to kick off once he knows you've tracked him down.'

'Do you know what's happening?' I asked, still keeping my voice low. 'Have you seen his mother?'

'Oh yes,' she said. 'Not half an hour ago. She's been back and gone straight out again. And she's fuming. They've apparently told her she's got to have some report or something done on her. Anyway, she's gone off to fetch her Carley from her mate's house, or so she tells me. She might just have gone off on the piss. That wouldn't surprise me. And then me laddo here turns up a couple of minutes later. And can't get in, of course. So I told him he could stop here for a bit. But I'm not happy about it. Not happy at all. If Karen finds out it was me called social services, she'll give me a right gob full …'

'So Jenson doesn't know anything about his mum coming back yet – what's been happening or what's going to happen? Did you tell him?'

'Good lord, no!' the woman told me. 'I'll leave all that to you lot, since you're here now.' She thought for a moment. 'But what about the social worker? Are you allowed to just take him, then? That's if he'll go with you anyway. No offence, but I doubt he will. Not without a fight.'

'The social worker is on her way,' I reassured her. 'And don't worry – we can leave her to deal with that side of things. I'm sure that between us we'll be able to get him to see reason, bless him. At least I hope so. The last thing she'll want is to have to drag him off against his will.'

The neighbour's expression changed a little. 'Poor lad,' she mused. 'He's a handful, I know. But it isn't right, is it?'

I shook my head, aware that I must be a bit circumspect. 'It's not good, for sure.'

'But you know,' she said, beckoning again that I should follow her into a different room, 'it's not his fault. It really isn't. Sometimes I see them together and I could weep for him, I really could. It's so obvious to everyone how different she treats them bairns. Blatant, it is. But it's always been that way – they probably told you all about it – since all that business with the little one ...' She shook her head sadly. 'Well, I don't care what the circumstances were, it's not right, it isn't – *anyone* can see that. Anyway, cup of tea, love? Might as well.'

My antennae twitching, I followed the woman into her small and pristine kitchen, and was just about to ask what she meant by 'all that business with the little one' when the poor lad himself exploded indoors through the back door, closely followed by a 'Heinz 57 varieties' kind of wiry-haired dog.

The dog leapt upon me with great enthusiasm – nothing remotely Alsatian-ish about it – but Jenson, understandably, stopped dead in his tracks. As well he might. I was obviously the last person he expected to see. But he gathered himself up defiantly. 'You're wasting your time,' he told me, scowling. 'I'm waiting for me mum and then I'm goin' home and you can't stop me.' He looked at his neighbour, then, presumably for corroboration.

But she was rescued from having to answer by a ring on her doorbell. Which she hurried off to answer.

'I'm not,' Jenson began. 'I'm not coming. You can't make me.' Then I watched his face fall further. 'Oh, God,' he said, in his world-weary voice, seeing Marie approaching down the hall. 'God! What is she doin' here?'

But Marie was impressive. While the neighbour – Mrs Clark – and I swapped phone numbers, in case it happened again, she calmly dealt with the situation like a pro. Within minutes Jenson had turned from a furious whirling dervish to, if not a happy, at least a calm and reasonably compliant bunny, prepared to accept, albeit grudgingly, the way things had to be.

'But when *can* I see her?' he asked mournfully, and my heart really went out to him. He'd gone to all that trouble (and what, come to think of it, had happened to his sister?) yet he'd missed his mum by minutes. And now he was being told he had to go straight back home with me. I think I would have kicked off, under the circumstances.

'Well,' Marie said, 'I will have to double-check this, obviously, but if you go with Casey now,' she glanced at me, 'then I think I'm pretty safe in promising that you will be able to see Mum after school tomorrow. Assuming you *go* to school, that is. And assuming you *stay* in school, as well. No running off, or Mum will just get into *more* trouble. D'you understand that?'

Jenson looked crushed suddenly, and I wished Marie hadn't placed such emphasis on the word 'more' there. Because Jenson had obviously leapt on it immediately. And I watched his eyes begin to fill with tears again. 'So is it my fault?' he said brokenly. 'Is she in trouble cos I ran off from school today – is that it?'

'Good lord, no!' Marie reassured him. 'No, not at *all*, Jenson.' She took his hand and squeezed it. 'Of course you *shouldn't* have run off – you know that, don't you?' Jenson nodded. 'You should have done as Casey and Mike said, shouldn't you?' He nodded again. 'But the judge decided what he decided before he even knew that. It's not your fault, Jenson. It was because Mum went on holiday, that was all. Because you're too young to be left – both of you; you and Carley are both too young, and she should have realised it wasn't appropriate to do that … that's all.'

Jenson turned to me now, wiping a sleeve across the end of his nose, obviously keen not to get either himself or his mother into any further trouble. 'I'm sorry for running off, Casey,' he said forlornly. Which made me want to scoop him up and hug him, but I resisted. It would probably just set him off crying all over again.

'That's okay, sweetie,' I said instead. 'You just gave us all a bit of a fright, that's all. No harm done.' I ruffled his hair. 'As long as you *don't do it again*, okay? Anyway, let's have this drink, shall we? Then we'll get you back to ours. Honestly, I can't believe you were all set to leave us without your new DS!'

Which raised a smile at last.

And Jenson did seem to cheer up as we headed back to our house, and delighted in explaining to me how he'd figured out his escape plan.

'I know the main gates get locked,' he explained. 'They have to do that cos of paedophiles and serial killers and that – so when it was lunchtime I went to the fence round the field. It's a long fence, and there's always bits where it's a bit broken and that. An' most of it leads on to a big road round the back, and it's good because the offices an' that are on the other side, so they can't see you. An' I found a place really easy, so that bit was okay …'

'And off you went.'

'No, I couldn'a gone then. Cos of the afternoon register. So I had to wait till I got a chance –'

'Which you were lucky to get, by all accounts.'

He looked sheepish. 'Yeah, well … an' so I had to take it, didn't I? An' then I just legged it over the field, took my school sweatshirt off, so no one would tell I was a school kid, and legged it all the way home.'

If I'd suppressed a smile at 'paedophiles and serial killers an' that', I was hard pushed to do so at his delightful 9-year-old reasoning that if he took off his sweatshirt no one would know he was a 'school kid'. An image came to mind, then, of an alternative universe. One in which there were two grades of child – the normal, school-going kind, and an underclass of other kids, who were occupied differently. Little chimney sweeps, vagabonds and Dickensian-style urchins, who roamed the streets when the rest were doing their sums. 'So,' I asked, 'what about your sister? What about Carley?'

The made him scowl. 'She an' Mum had already gone – I *knew* they would! I just knew it!'

'Gone where?'

Jenson shrugged. 'Round Gary's, most probly. I bet Carley didn't think I'd do it. But I *did*!'

I decided not to probe further into the machinations of Jenson's family. Best not to inflame things further and get him all wound up again. But one thing was for sure – it didn't augur well for the outcome, in terms of getting Jenson home again. I had just the one impression of his mum so far – irresponsible. No, actually, two. Irresponsible and neglectful. And just what was the business with 'the little one' all about?

I pulled up outside the house and asked Jenson what he'd like for tea. I would find out soon enough, no doubt. Or wouldn't. Either way, what would be would be.

Because I hadn't been expecting to hear anything from anyone again till the following morning, when the house phone rang later I was sure that this time it had to be my mother. I hadn't even heard it, in fact, because I was clearing up the dinner things while listening to my favourite fifties and sixties golden-oldie radio station. As this was generally the signal for anyone else in the house to scarper, I whacked it up loud and invariably sang along.

So the first I knew of the call was when Jenson appeared in the kitchen doorway, just in time to catch my interpretation of a jaunty Sandie Shaw number.

'Oh!' I said, seeing him and turning the radio down. There was something of a shocked expression on his face, and I felt slightly self-conscious to have been caught jigging around – or what did they call it now, throwing shapes? – in my kitchen. And judging by the way he was looking at me, so did he. 'Sorry, love,' I added, wiping my hands and taking the phone from him. He gave me a priceless head shake and returned to watching TV with Mike.

'Casey?' It wasn't my mum. It was John Fulshaw. 'Sorry to call you at this hour,' he said. 'I know I'm making something of a habit of bothering you just lately. I was going to leave a message on your mobile. But then I realised I'm going to be tied up in a meeting till lunchtime tomorrow, and I really need to run this by you as a matter of urgency.'

My ears pricked up. Did this mean Jenson was about to leave us? Or had the situation worsened in some way? But he'd used the words 'run by you', which didn't seem to fit either.

'What's happened?' I said, intrigued.

'Nothing's happened exactly. It's just that we have a bit of a dilemma. We have this boy, you see, Georgie –'

'Another boy?' I was confused now. And then something struck me. Was this something to do with Jenson's family? Was this the little one the neighbour had attested to?

'Another boy,' John confirmed. 'To be honest, we have had you and Mike in mind for him for a while now.'

'Oh!' I said, re-jigging my train of thought completely. This was obviously a different boy. A potential foster placement. 'So he's one of the ones you mentioned the other day, is he?'

'Exactly,' confirmed John. 'Except it's looking like we need to place him sooner rather than later. He has his problems, Casey – this is going to be something a bit different for you.'

'In what way?' I wanted to know. I was even more intrigued now, prickle on the back of the neck intrigued.

'He has a degree of autism, to be precise about it. A fair degree of it. Which presents its own challenges, as I'm sure you're aware.'

Which I knew it did and would. But there was obviously more to it than that. I was most interested to know why he'd been placed in care. 'What's his family situation?'

'There is none. No family. He's been in children's homes since he was a toddler. Very young mother. Still in her mid-teens. Simply couldn't cope with him. And, from what I've seen of the file – to be honest, I've barely scratched the surface – the family weren't supportive. Well, you can imagine the scenario, can't you? Without that kind of support it must have been a big ask for her. So, sadly, the girl put him into care herself.'

I took a moment to digest that, and to wonder how it must have felt. What a tragedy, for all concerned. 'Oh, John, that's so sad ...'

'Isn't it? But also a fact of life, unfortunately. But don't run away with the idea that this is a kid with a load of baggage. He's been in the same children's home since he was 2 and knows no other life. And is a contented little soul, by all accounts. Well, was. That happy state of affairs might not continue. As I say, the home's closing down, and he needs a new one pronto. They've been looking for a long-term foster home for him for a while now.'

'What, as in *us*?' Long-term foster care wasn't in our remit. Our job was to provide short placements – no more than nine months or so, usually, to set the behaviourally challenged kids up so they were *fit* for long-term fostering.

'No, no,' John said. 'That was never the plan, obviously. He's 9 – same age as Jenson – and he needs somewhere he can stay till he's 18. In an ideal world, at any rate. So in the meantime we'd earmarked you and Mike as perhaps the perfect interim placement. With your understanding of Asperger's – and I know it's not anywhere near the same degree of disability – we thought you'd be better placed to take care of him than most. And best of all, he's local – and we'd like to keep him local, if at all possible. It will be enough of an upheaval leaving his home as it is, without changing his whole environment as well ...'

'And you don't think another children's home is the answer?'

'I wish! Because he is perfectly settled. Funny, isn't it? That the very things that make children's homes less than ideal for most kids mean they're perfect places for children like Georgie. He loves the routine, loves the privacy, and loves the institutionalised nature of it. And he hates change, obviously. But since this whole drive to try and move kids into family situations ... Sounds crazy, but they're becoming as rare as hens' teeth. Ones that can accommodate a child like Georgie, at any rate.'

Which was true. Children's homes had become deeply unpopular in recent years. And with good reason – the statistics regarding the life chances of kids who were raised in them made for depressing reading in the extreme. But John was spot on – a child such as he was describing, with their complex needs and lack of emotional challenges, could often thrive in such an institutionalised environment. Plus he had obviously never known a family of his own.

'So,' I said, 'what's the matter of urgency in this equation?'

'The home is closing imminently – they've moved it forward a couple of weeks. Which means that, ideally, we need to place him now, this minute. Bless him – he's the only kid left in there, Casey.'

My heart melted, hearing that. The poor kid. He must be scared witless with all that upheaval going on around him. And to be the only child left – it must be horrible. And, of course, I thought immediately of Kieron.

'How severe is his autism,' I asked John, 'in practical terms?'

'Well, I remember reading that he's in mainstream school, supported by a specialist teaching assistant, so that says a lot. And knowing you and Mike, I'm sure there's nothing you can't handle. I can call in tomorrow, if you like, and we can run through the paperwork in more detail, but I thought that with Jenson probably off your hands within the week it might be doable. Just a short overlap with the both of them ...'

'It's okay,' I said, 'you don't need to do a big sell. Of course we'll take him, John.'

He chuckled. 'Hadn't you better speak to Mike first?'

So I did speak to Mike, and, of course, he did his usual Mike thing.

'Are you sure you can manage both of them?' he said. 'It could potentially be quite challenging. If this kid's used to being alone, and being in a home, he might find that difficult.'

'Yes,' I said, 'but I'm sure there won't be anything that'll faze me. Not with a couple of 9-year-olds.'

Mike gave me one of his old-fashioned looks. He knew as well as I that he could name at least two boys we'd fostered – no, three, come to think of it – who fitted that description. And there had been *plenty* to faze me. To faze both of us.

'And remember,' he said, playing up to his established role of calmer-downer, 'autism is not the same as Asperger's, Case.'

'I know that!'

'And what if they don't get on? You've considered that scenario, have you?'

'Of course I have,' I countered. 'And we can cross that bridge when we come to it. Anyway, why must you always think of the worst?'

'I'm glad you mentioned that,' Mike said, 'because it might be a bridge we have to cross. Suppose Jenson turns out to be with us for longer than we thought? I'm just trying to make you see all the angles, love, that's all.'

Which was fine. That was his job, and it was good that I had him to do it. But, at the same time, I had my job. To look always on the bright side. And, being well practised now in such situations, I had answers good and ready for all his supplementary questions as well.

'After all,' I said gaily, when Mike finally allowed me to call John back, 'how difficult can two little boys be?'

Chapter 8

'Say yes and worry about the details later' is probably a good mantra for life generally. But not in every case, perhaps. Maybe, sometimes, it *is* the fools who tend to rush in. Had I been one, I wondered, having been so quick to rush in here? Because pleased though I was to be able to make John's day – and I clearly had – almost as soon as I started speaking to him about Georgie I began to feel anxious as well.

He had explained that, in this case, a prior visit would be counterproductive, not only because logistically it would be difficult to arrange at such short notice, but also because with change being so upsetting for the boy it was in his best interests if they left it till the last minute.

'So I was wondering,' John was saying, 'if you could email me a few photos of the family. Ideally in some home locations, so he can get a look at the environment as well. We've got you and Mike's mug shots on file somewhere, of course, but a few family snaps – of the whole clan, ideally; everyone he's likely to come into contact with – would be a good and less unsettling introduction.'

I agreed that I would. 'And at the same time I'll pop some notes over for you,' he said. 'I've got a few already and I'm pleased to be able to tell you that he'll be arriving with a comprehensive care plan.'

He chortled, having said this, and I could hear the irony in his voice, because that would be a *very* welcome change. How many times had we taken on children with almost nothing about their history to go on? Too many. Oh, the notes were always 'on their way' or 'in the process of getting updated' but more often than not they simply failed to materialise – or, even if they did, came in such dribs and drabs that by the time we read that this or that event or incident had happened we didn't *need* telling – because we'd already seen it in action for ourselves.

But, thankful as I was that this time we'd have a bit more to go on than just a couple of measly A4 sheets of not-very-much, it was still sinking in that we might be biting off more than we could chew here. For starters, the poor child would probably be terrified. Would I have the skills to be able to comfort him? Would I be able to even understand what he needed?

I mentally shook myself. Of course I would. And if I didn't, I could learn. After all, I might feel slightly unequal to the task, but what were the alternatives? Someone who'd probably feel every bit as much out of their depth, but who didn't even have the benefit of being close to Georgie's school. Or, worse still, the prospect of being pushed from pillar to post in a series of short respite placements.

No, we'd be fine, I told myself, and told John as well. 'But what about Jenson?' I finished. 'How d'you want me to play it with him?'

John seemed surprised. 'Oh, I shouldn't worry about that aspect,' he said. 'In all likelihood they'll only have to rub along for a couple of days.'

He probably didn't realise the irony of those words any more than I did. Rubbing along, after all, meant one thing – friction.

Relaying all this to Mike after Jenson had gone to bed, I was pleased to find myself beginning to feel as relaxed about that aspect of it as John had. 'So I'm not going to make a big thing of it,' I told him as I climbed into bed. 'I'll just run it by him over breakfast, I think. He might even find it a welcome distraction. You know – divert him from fretting about his mum.'

And I was of exactly the same mindset the following morning, which had dawned to be another beautiful spring day. So much so that I even decided we'd have our breakfast on the patio: boiled eggs, which I was just bringing to the table when Jenson appeared.

'Oh,' he said, intrigued to see the outside table laid. 'We eating out here then?'

'Indeed we are,' I answered, pouring him a tumbler of orange juice. 'It's called *al fresco*.'

'Al what?'

'*Al fresco*,' I repeated. 'It's Italian. Italian for eating outside. Anyway, crack on,' I quipped, as he reached for his teaspoon. 'I'll go and fetch my coffee and the toast and cut you up some soldiers.'

Jenson grinned. 'Brill,' he said. 'Mum always makes us soldiers. You haven't forgotten you're going to ring up today, have you?'

'No,' I called back, as I went back inside to fetch the toast for him. 'Soon as I've dropped you off, don't worry.'

He'd taken the top off his egg by the time I got back outside, and was waiting patiently for the bread to dip into it. That was one thing, I mused, as I cut toast into fingers. At least she bothered enough to make him soldiers.

'Oh, and by the way,' I said, as I passed the hot buttered toast to him, 'I have some news.'

'You have?'

'Not about you. It's some other news. You know you're only going to be with us for a short time?'

Jenson nodded, and had the good grace not to say 'thank goodness'. 'Well,' I said, 'I've been speaking to our boss, John, on the phone. And he's asked us if we'll take on our next placement early.'

Jenson looked confused. Of course, I thought. Silly me. He wouldn't understand that concept, would he? 'The next child,' I explained, 'that we're going to be having longer term. Do you remember me telling you that that was what we usually did? Have children for a few months to do our special training programme? Well, this is the next child we're due to have, and as we're going to have him a little early, it means that for a few days at least we'll have both of you living with us.'

Jenson digested this along with a mouthful of egg.

'So it's a boy?' he said.

'It is.'

'How old is he?'

'Almost the same age as you.'

'Older or younger?'

'I don't know. All I know is that he's 9.'

Jenson considered this as he ate. 'An' is he gonna share my room with me?'

'No, no. He'll have his own bedroom. We wouldn't expect you to share a room.'

His eyes narrowed. 'Yeah, but will I have to share my DS with him?'

'Heavens, no. That's yours, Jenson! So, no – not unless you want to let him. But I imagine he'll have his own toys, don't you?'

Jenson continued to dip toast into the top of his egg. 'What's his name?'

'Georgie.'

'Georgie?' His brows furrowed. 'As in Georgie-*ee*?'

'I know – it does sound a little bit like a girl's name, doesn't it? But it isn't. It's –'

Jenson had paused with a piece of toast halfway to his mouth, dripping yolk.

'Careful,' I said. 'Don't want to get egg yolk on your school trousers.' But he didn't seem to be aware of the toast now.

'Georg*ie*?' he said again. 'Georgie who? What's his surname?'

'Umm,' I thought, trying to recall. 'Umm, let me see … Georgie Smart, I think. Yes, that's it.'

'Georgie Smart?' he spluttered, dropping the toast back onto his plate now. 'Georgie *Smart*?'

Yes, I said, surprised. 'Why? Do you know him?'

'*Know* him?' he said, looking mortified. 'Of *course* I know him! *Everybody* knows him! He's a dummy! He's not Georgie Smart, either – he's Georgie Not-so-smart!'

Well, what a turn up, I thought. 'Jenson,' I said. 'Does Georgie go to your sch—'

But he wasn't listening. He was too busy looking mortified. 'Are you saying *he's* going to live *here*? Here, in this *house*?'

I nodded. 'Yes,' I said. 'Yes he is. So he goes to your school then?'

Jenson groaned. 'But he's such a *retard*! All the other kids will take the piss! He can't live here!'

I needed to rein this in. 'Jenson, it's not a case of "can't". He *is*. And I'd be grateful if you'd stop making such unkind comments about him.'

'But he *is*,' he persisted. 'An' he's scary. He says all this weird shit –'

'Jenson!'

'But he *does*. He's just crazy. He can't come here. No way.'

He was pushing his chair back now, shaking his head in disbelief. 'Jenson,' I began.

'I can't *believe* you're doing this to me,' he said wretchedly. Then he stomped off back inside the house.

Great, I thought, pushing my own chair back and following. Shouldn't John have known something like this? No, perhaps not, I conceded. I really couldn't expect every tiny detail of every child to pop into his brain every minute of every day, could I? It probably wouldn't have occurred to him to even think about it. There must have been any one of a dozen primary schools either boy could have gone to. It was a big area, well populated. What were the chances? But I hadn't thought about it either, more was the pity.

By now I could hear Jenson banging around upstairs, and it occurred to me that potentially I had something of a situation here. He was off to school now – Georgie's school – after all. Their paths might cross. He might say something. The complications were stacking up.

'Jenson,' I said, putting on my stern face as he stomped back down the stairs. 'Listen, I know this isn't ideal for you – I doubt it is for Georgie either. In fact, I know it's not – but it's what's happening, and I'd like to think you can be mature enough to make the best of it. Who knows, once you get to know him a little, you might even find something positive to be able to say to him, mightn't you? And as we both know, it's only likely to be for a few days. Okay?'

Jenson scowled, but at least managed to produce a grudging nod, though I was once again concerned that it was only because he'd already decided to do another runner back home. 'Anyway,' I continued briskly, 'you will in all probability be able to see Mum today, so that's good, isn't it? So be sure to be ready when I come to collect you this afternoon, because if you *are* seeing her today I will be driving you to go and see her. Down in town –' I made sure to emphasise that bit. With any luck, that should discourage him from absconding.

'And as far as Georgie goes,' I finished, handing him his backpack, 'I'd be grateful if you don't say anything to him about what's happening, okay? Because he doesn't know yet, and it will make him agitated, you understand?'

Jenson shouldered his backpack and regaled me with one of his less lovely expressions. 'Oh, don't worry,' he said. 'There's no way I'll be speaking to him – because he's a *freak!*'

Great, I thought again. And a very happy Monday to you all.

I was at least partly reassured after visiting Andrea Cappleman. It may or may not have been as a result of Jenson absconding from school on the previous Friday, but when she promised me she would ensure Jenson and Georgie didn't come into contact with one another before the end of the week I knew I could trust her to see to it that they didn't. Though I still felt another stab of anxiety. If Georgie was viewed as dispiritingly as he obviously was in some quarters, there was still a fair chance he'd get wind that something was going on. Much as I wished I could feel differently, I had enough experience around kids to know that Jenson would find it almost impossible not to share his news with all his peers – which meant it would probably be all around the school by lunchtime.

But I couldn't dwell on that; my job was to deal with the fall-out later. And in the meantime I had things to do myself.

John was apologetic that he hadn't twigged about the schools being the same. But I wasn't hard on him anyway, because it didn't really make a difference. And, actually, I thought, as I disconnected from him, being exposed more intimately to Georgie might prove a useful learning tool for young Jenson. So much prejudice stems from fear – that was a well-documented fact. And who knew? Perhaps exposure to a 'different' child like Georgie would form the basis of a useful bit of personal development.

If a short-lived one. My next call was to Marie Bateman, and I was pleased to hear that Jenson would indeed be seeing his mum.

'Not today, though, I'm afraid,' she said. 'Which I know is going to disappoint him. But I just can't squeeze it into my schedule this afternoon. I wish I could, but you just can't get a quart into a pint pot – and you know the sort of workloads people like you and I have all too well! Tomorrow, though. Tomorrow after school.'

'What do you want me to do then?' I asked, understanding where she was coming from re the workload. I felt for her. At least I didn't have to spend my days in interminable meetings these days.

'Oh, nothing. Nothing at all,' she said. 'I'll come and pick him up after straight after school, if that's okay.'

'Oh,' I said. 'You sure? That would be brilliant. It would give me a chance to get some paperwork done. Not to mention start preparing the spare room ready for Georgie.'

'Absolutely,' she said. 'Though would that you could. No, that's the point. Until things are sorted, they have to be supervised contact visits. Couple of things have come up that need to be gone into. So they'll be doing a full assessment of both Karen and the boyfriend.'

'Anything I should know about?' I asked, my ears immediately pricking up, recalling 'all that business with the little one'. I was used to fostering policies, and information being given to us on a need-to-know basis, but it was often the case that social workers assumed I already knew something from my link worker and vice versa.

'Nothing we can talk about yet,' she answered guardedly. 'We just need to dig a little deeper on a couple of matters so that we can satisfy the court's criteria before sending the kids home. We'll keep you informed, of course.'

'But you're still expecting that they're going home?' I asked her.

'I've not heard anything to the contrary,' she answered, equally vaguely.

Oh well, I thought, as I put down the phone on her. *Let's just hope they get it sorted out sooner rather than later.* And in the meantime I'd just have to deal with whatever challenges this novel situation decided to throw at me, wouldn't I?

I just hoped I wouldn't need a crash helmet …

Chapter 9

Jenson was like a cat on hot bricks the following afternoon, waiting for the social worker to arrive. He'd been so excited at the thought of seeing his mum again that he'd even been effusive about letting me know how good he'd been in not saying anything to Georgie.

'I saw him today again and everything,' he said. 'Coming into the dinner hall with his special teacher woman, an' I never said a word to him, Casey. Not *nothing*. I just turned my head away an' ignored him.'

For all that I noted how he managed to make 'special' sound like a dirty word, I was really pleased to hear this. He obviously *could* be a good boy – though I pointed out that Georgie's special teacher woman would have actually been a teaching assistant, and that lots of kids got help from these kinds of teachers, so that they could get the best out of what the regular teachers told them.

And when Marie's car pulled up, it was all I could do to stop Jenson flying straight out of the house without a backward glance.

'Oh, God!' he moaned, as I clamped a restraining hand on his shoulder. 'We're gonna be late if she starts gabbing with you, Casey!'

'Less of the cheek,' I admonished, as Marie walked up the path. 'All set to go?' I asked her. 'I certainly know someone who is.'

Marie nodded. 'I'll have him back in a couple of hours,' she promised. 'Is that all right?'

It was more than all right. It was already Tuesday afternoon and I hadn't yet made any preparations for Georgie's arrival. He was due at teatime on Thursday and I'd not even made a start on his room yet. After phoning Mike and asking if he'd bring some fish and chips home for tea, I decided to go up and attack it with my Marigolds.

The pink room wasn't ideal but, as I'd already explained to John, it would only be temporary. Once Jenson had left, I'd simply move Georgie into the blue room. Still, I did chastise myself a little for acting in such haste over the colour schemes. I thought I'd been quite clever at the time. After all, my reasoning had gone, it would always be one or the other: they'd either send me a boy – blue room – or they'd send me a girl – pink room – so at the time it seemed the perfect way to go. That it had never occurred to me that I might be sent a pair of brothers or sisters now seemed quite loopy – I'd had siblings before, hadn't I?

But no matter, I thought, as I trotted up the stairs with my cleaning things – he'd be okay in there for a short while – might even want to stay in there, in fact. Given the way his mind worked, he might not even care about such things.

Looking at the extreme pinkness, however – particularly of the curtains and bedding – I did toy with opting for the other spare room instead. But that made no sense. It had a double bed, for starters, which was useful if family came to stay, so it would be a shame to limit that option, and it also looked a bit fusty, dominated, as is was, by a gigantic oak wardrobe that we had somehow inherited from my grand-mother. My parents had stored it for us for several years (it was apparently too valuable a family heirloom to put on eBay) but since our move six months back they had decreed that since we now had room for it they could finally get shot of it, to make way for something more modern.

No, the pink room it had to be, so I set about stripping the bed and replacing the butterflies-and-daisies duvet cover with something more neutral.

That done, I then sorted out a few toys, books and games and then, after giving the room a quick buff and polish, went downstairs to print out all the information John had emailed me about Georgie, so I could have a good read with a cup of coffee while it was quiet.

While there's no single behaviour that is 'typical' of autism, there are several behaviours that are more frequently found than others. And it seems Georgie had several of these. For example, he had something called echolalia. This basically meant the parrot-like repetition of words and phrases he might hear. He might come out with a string of sentences from a television programme, for example, or continually repeat something a teacher or parent might say. Almost always, these speech patterns would be non-contextual, too, i.e. they would come out completely randomly, often far removed from where he heard them, which was why – and this was true of my experience of autistic kids in school – children like Georgie would become such easy targets for bullying.

He also apparently – again like lots of kids with autism – had a marked lack of empathy. This meant he struggled to perceive the emotional state of others, which, again, made relationships with peers challenging.

Other aspects were pretty much as I'd expected them to be. A long list of likes and even longer list of dislikes. And with the latter, it wasn't just a case of a simple dislike – if something happened or was given to him that was on the list of dislikes, it could provoke an extreme emotional reaction.

I was on surer ground with all his rituals – since, to a lesser degree, that was something important to my Kieron – but I sighed to see it emphasised how much he found human contact painful. This would be a child who'd react adversely to that most basic human drive – to cuddle, to hold hands, to be kissed better.

It was all quite sobering food for thought. When I had worked with kids like Georgie in the past, it had been in a school setting; a place consistent in its own rituals, rules and routines. Which made it straightforward, and also, in terms of human contact, not all that stressful – in school there was a distance; a fair degree of personal space. But in a home setting – a place of warmth, spontaneity and affection – such boundaries would feel very strange.

At the bottom of the notes were some contact details for Georgie's social worker – a Mr Harry Bird. And also a note to say he'd be getting in touch by phone on Thursday morning, just to talk through final details, answer any of my questions, and tell me what I could expect when Georgie first arrived.

'It all sounds terribly serious,' I told Mike over the promised fish and chips an hour later. 'Like we're taking temporary responsibility for some rare species of animal, or a crucial component for some space rocket or something.'

Mike laughed. 'It's just a child, Case,' he said. 'Just another kid. You'll be fine ...'

'I'm not so sure,' I said, dousing my chips in vinegar. 'I think it's going to be a lot more difficult than we imagined. It's certainly going to take a lot of patience.'

'Calm,' Mike said.

'Calm?'

'Calm – that was our watchword, remember? When Kieron was little. D'you remember how we used to say it all the time? Like the paediatrician told us?' He chuckled again. 'Though, fair point – there *is* young Jenson to consider. I'm not sure Jenson knows the meaning of the word calm.'

I acknowledged this with a frown. Of course Jenson didn't do calm. My impression, brief though it was, was that calm was a commodity in short supply in his life. If we were choosing 'c' words, chaos seemed to fit better.

'Impossible,' I said.

'No,' said Mike.' Not impossible, love. Not for a super-mum like you. Just challenging. And how many times have you told me how much you relish challenges?'

He was grinning. 'Shut your face,' I told him sharply.

When Jenson arrived home he was full of smiles and full of beans. Which was gratifying to see. You never knew with parental contact visits. Sometimes they panned out. Very often they were a disaster. And given that there was still no date fixed for him and his sister to return home, seeing his mum might have actually proved distressing.

But this was evidently not the case. He just seemed genuinely thrilled to have seen her. 'She's got a right tan on, Casey. You should see her! An' guess what? Her an' Gary only got engaged when they were in Spain! She said he fell for her hook and line and what's the other thing, Marie?'

'Hook, line and sinker,' Marie finished for him. Then glanced at me. 'So all's well in Karen-land ...'

'Karen-land,' Jenson quipped. 'That's cool that is. I'll have to remember that for next time.'

I looked at Marie enquiringly.

'Which will be Saturday,' she clarified. 'If that works for you. Pick him up around nine thirty. The plan at the moment is to go bowling. Then lunch – I think we decided on pizza, didn't we, Jenson?' Jenson nodded. 'And then back to you around three, I imagine.'

I agreed that would be good for us – mainly it would give me a big chunk of time alone with Georgie – and while Jenson went off upstairs to change out of his school uniform I took the opportunity to ask Marie if he'd mentioned anything about the fact that Georgie was moving in.

'Not a word,' she said. 'To be honest, he wouldn't have had much of a chance anyway. That woman can talk for Britain – and it's all about her, of course. How great her holiday was, how excited she was about her engagement ... And you should have seen her – done up as if she was planning on going straight on to a night club. Skirt up to here, enough make-up to restock Boots – honestly, I know it's unprofessional to judge by appearances, but between you and me I wasn't very impressed. Barely a word about what the kids had been up to, or how sorry she was about the situation ...' She sighed. And, mentally, I sighed with her.

'So sad, isn't it?' I said. 'You'd think, given the little time she had to spend with him, that she'd at least have made the effort to make a bit of a fuss.'

'I know,' agreed Marie, 'but what surprised me most was that Jenson didn't seem in the slightest bit bothered by it. He was just over the moon to be even in her company.'

Which was perfectly natural but felt even more sad. No child should feel so lacking in maternal love that they had to cling on pathetically for ever tiny morsel of affection that was on offer.

But both in my current job and also in the one before it I had come across a depressingly large minority of mothers who were so wrapped up in their own lives that they couldn't see for looking where the trials of their children's lives were concerned. It wasn't rocket science to work out that there was generally a reason for kids displaying challenging behaviours.

Still, I thought, Jenson was in a good place at the moment, which was all we could ask for. I just hoped it would last.

Mike was able to leave work early in preparation for Georgie's arrival the following afternoon, which I was grateful for. He'd worked for the same company for years, and had always been loyal and hard working, so, since we'd begun fostering, they'd always been great about those times when he needed a little flexibility. Which he did, as even though the house was entirely shipshape he knew I'd have my usual last-minute flap about dust. But when he walked through the front door I could see something was missing.

'Mike,' I groaned, 'don't tell me you forgot to get the flowers.'

I had texted him earlier to get some from the supermarket on the way home, but it seemed he'd forgotten.

'Love, this is a 9-year-old boy,' he argued reasonably. 'You think he's even going to notice whether there are flowers in the house?'

'But they make the house smell nice,' I whined as I followed him into the kitchen. 'And, besides, I've never met this new social worker, have I?'

Mike laughed then. 'Ah, of course,' he said. 'That's what this is all about then, is it?' He glanced out of the patio doors. 'All right,' he said. 'You put the kettle on. I'll go down the garden and see what I can find.'

In that respect, we'd been lucky. We'd moved into the house just before Christmas, with little idea what surprises lay ready under the ground. And we'd been rewarded, by first crocuses and daffodils and tulips, and now a wonderful array of perennial flowers – including peonies and lupins – and best of all, a couple of elderly but healthy rose bushes, all of which, by some miracle, had managed to avoid being beheaded by flying footballs.

I had just grabbed a vase for the half a dozen lemony roses he'd cut for me, when I spied a man and a boy coming up the path. The man – Harry Bird, I assumed – seemed exactly as I had pictured him: mid- or late fifties, greying hair, unfussy glasses, well-worn suit. He'd already called me that morning, just as he'd promised, with the reassuring news that Georgie seemed reasonably understanding of what was happening and had apparently taken great interest in the photographs. He'd been particularly mesmerised, Mr Bird had told me, with my black hair. The boy himself, who was wearing the same school uniform as Jenson's, was clutching a round silver tin. He looked about average height and build for his age – a little more robustly built than Jenson – though I couldn't see his face as he had his chin tucked firmly into his chest. I couldn't miss his hair, though. He had the most beautiful, shoulder-length mass of blond curls. I'd never seen anything quite like it – well, apart from on rock stars. It was stunning.

Still holding the vase of flowers, I opened the front door to greet them. Harry Bird grinned and extended a hand to shake mine. As my right arm was still wrapped around the vase, I made a quick transfer. 'Casey Watson,' I said. 'Sorry – excuse the roses.'

The little boy up to now hadn't looked anywhere other than down, where he now seemed to be making a close inspection of my gravelled front garden. But now he raised his head and, looking at no one in particular, said: 'Rose Marion Tyler, species: human, home planet: earth, 48 Bucknall House, the Powell estate, London SE15 7GO.'

I smiled at Georgie, feeling glad that I'd been prepped about this. And was careful not to touch him as I ushered them both inside. No pat on the shoulder. No ruffling of that gorgeous hair.

Hmm, though, I thought as Mike led them into the kitchen diner. Rose Marion Tyler. Where had I heard that name before?

Chapter 10

Harry Bird supplied the answer to my unspoken question. '*Doctor Who*,' he said, putting down his tatty leather brief-case. 'Georgie's a big fan, aren't you, lad?'

There was clearly a rapport between the two of them, I noticed, because he then leaned towards Georgie and, in an almost faultless replica of the fabled killing machines, stuck an arm out and growled, 'Ex-ter-min-ate!'

Georgie looked up and then back to his palms, which he'd cupped, as if holding an imaginary crystal ball. 'Dalek,' he said. 'A mutated organism with a polycarbide mechanical casing. Seeks universal domination. Ex-ter-min-ate.'

'Wow,' said Mike, as he switched on the kettle. 'Impressive! I used to love *Doctor Who* when I was a kid too. D'you want to take your coat off, Georgie?'

Georgie nodded, though, as we'd been led to expect, he didn't make eye contact with Mike as he removed it. He then carefully folded it and scanned the room for a place to put it down.

'Over there, love,' I said, pointing to the slim cupboard in the kitchen. 'That's where we keep all our everyday coats and shoes. And while you're doing that I'll make you a glass of juice, shall I?'

Again, there was no direct response but as Georgie walked across to put his coat away he began shaking his head from side to side.

'Milk, please, for Georgie,' Harry quickly translated. 'If that's okay … Georgie likes to drink milk. He doesn't like juice. In fact he … well, once we sit down for a chat it will all be a bit easier. That okay?'

'Of course,' I said, feeling pleased that – from first impressions anyway – here was a social worker who knew his charge well. As he would; he might have been with him from the outset – probably had. Which was a big plus. Because right now I was bewildered. So having someone on hand who really knew what made him tick would be a huge benefit for all of us.

'You seem to know him extremely well,' I said. 'It's good that we've got someone who has a handle on all the ins and outs. Makes a refreshing change, in fact.'

'Not for long, I'm afraid,' Harry said with a sigh. 'I'm due to retire soon, and Georgie is the last child on my case load. I'd have gone already, between you and me, but I agreed to wait until we had him settled before I hung up my briefcase.'

So that was that bubble burst right away. Harry went on to explain that a new worker would be assigned in due course, but that it might take a while as they would need to get the match right. It obviously needed someone who was conversant with the type of problems Georgie faced, which wouldn't be the easiest thing in the world.

But it would be silly to stress about the future at this point. All that mattered was what was happening now. And that meant the business of Georgie living with Mike and me, and Jenson, who, as if on cue, chose that precise moment to come in. He greeted us, rather charmingly, with a huge belch.

'Jenson!' I admonished, mortified.

'Pardon me!' he said, grinning. 'All right there, Georgie Porgie?' he asked. 'You see me in school earlier? I seen you. Seen you coming out of your *special* room.'

He'd managed to load the word 'special' with all the sarcasm he could muster, and once again I winced.

'Jenson,' I said again, 'if you remember, I did ask you to give us a bit of privacy while we got all this sorted out. So would you please either go back into the living room or upstairs to your bedroom. I'll call you down as soon as we're done, okay?'

But before he could answer, Georgie – who'd now walked back to where Harry was – was once again shaking his head and cupping his hands. 'He kissed the girls and made them cry,' he said. 'Not Georgie. Georgie did not do this.'

I glared at Jenson, who quickly scarpered, his bit of mischief over with, while Mike set a tumbler of milk down on the table for Georgie.

'Sorry about that,' he said to Harry, as he passed round all our coffees. 'They know each other from school – as you probably know.' Harry nodded. 'So it's obviously all a bit "I'm the top dog here because I got here first" right now. Nothing to worry about, though. We'll soon have that sorted. It'll be okay, mate,' he finished, looking at Georgie.

'No worries at all,' Harry said cheerfully, directing Georgie to his drink. 'Actually, if it's all right with you two, I think now might be a good time to get Georgie settled in front of the telly. There's a quiz show on shortly that he's rather keen on – *Countdown*. Aren't you, mate?' he said to Georgie. 'And he's cracking at it, too. Certainly seems to beat most of the contestants. And he's particularly quick at the conundrums.'

Again, he looked at Georgie, and I saw the merest hint of a smile cross Georgie's lips. But, just as was sometimes the case with tiny babies when it came to smiles, was I just seeing what I wanted to see? For this kid was a conundrum himself. He was clearly aware of his environment – taking in, and responding to, what was going on around him – but he seemed reliant upon others taking control. I realised I had barely scratched the surface with my research into autism, and something else – that I really liked Harry Bird. I loved this gentle, down-to-earth kind of social worker, period. The kind that was motivated by a genuine love of kids; the roll-your-sleeves-up-and-get-on-with-it kind of social worker.

Which made it doubly sad that he'd be leaving so soon. But not that much of a shock, once I thought about it. His type of social worker was such a rarity. And, currently, as well, a dying breed. The case loads social workers were expected to deal with these days meant that it was really hard for them to get to know the children in their care. They knew them superficially, of course – and perhaps sufficiently to do their best for them – but a bond such as I was witnessing between Georgie and Harry was a rare thing, and would only become rarer.

But there was nothing we could do about it, so it was silly to be sentimental. And with both boys sorted, Mike and Harry and I went back to the kitchen and got down to business. The tatty briefcase (another mark of a career social worker of long standing) was opened to reveal what was probably the fattest manila file of case notes I'd yet seen. Which wasn't that hard, given we so often seemed to be going into placements half-blind – but even so, for a kid who'd spent almost all his life in one care home, there were screeds and screeds of notes.

And I made more of them, scribbling furiously on my usual pad as Harry went through Georgie's routines in detail – adhering to these was key, he said, to avoiding too many 'freak-outs'. It was also interesting to note that, unusual for a child in care, Georgie had almost no belongings.

'He can't handle too much choice,' Harry explained, which took me straight away back to Kieron, who would also 'freak out', albeit mostly quietly, if bombarded with too much choice. 'So we've learned over the years that it's best to keep things simple,' Harry explained. 'For example, he has just the seven sets of winter clothes and the seven sets of summer clothes – any more than this and he'll simply refuse to get dressed. Same goes with footwear; one pair of indoor shoes, one pair of outdoor shoes, one pair for special occasions – no more, no less.'

'What about toys?' I asked. 'Does he have a special one? And are there any particular games he likes playing?'

Harry shook his head. 'Georgie doesn't really do toys, Casey. Never has. What tends to happen is that he'll develop attachments. Could be anything – and it's usually something completely random and obscure. When that happens, he becomes completely absorbed in whatever it is. Right now it's stones.'

'Stones?' Mike asked.

'Stones,' Harry confirmed. 'Stones of all sorts. Pebbles, bits of brick, rough, smooth, whatever. And we can't pinpoint what the attraction is because his collection is so varied. Shiny stones, smooth stones, rough stones, chipped stones … All different colours and textures – who knows what's going on?'

'He has a collection?' I asked, remembering the small silver tin, which Georgie had taken with him into the living room.

But it wasn't the tin, apparently. That was just for the most special stones. The main collection was still in the car. 'Shall we go out and get his things in?' Harry suggested. 'Mike, perhaps you could give me a hand with his cases. And I'll show you his collections box as well.'

We filed outside. 'Like I was saying,' Harry said, as he clicked the remote to release the car boot, 'it's stones at the moment but it could change at any time. Last year it was labels off of food tins – he had hundreds of the bloody things.' He chuckled. 'You can imagine how well that one went down at the home, can't you? He'd go on these sorties into the pantry and strip them off all the cans. Poor cook never knew what she'd be dishing up for tea till she'd opened one ...'

We both laughed but, as Mike helped Harry in with Georgie's things, I felt a twinge of apprehension about what we were taking on. Memories of Kieron's childhood flooded my mind now – all those little things I'd all but forgotten, like how upset he'd get when we'd go to a shop and he'd want to spend his pocket money, yet would be paralysed by indecision and distress. He'd invariably end up just copying Riley and spending his pennies on whatever she did, whether it was something he liked or not. What a learning curve that had been. And how much of a bigger one might *this* be? Once again I felt relieved to have some-one like Harry on hand to advise us, but even so this really felt like a journey into the unknown.

Georgie's collections tin was a large silver one, embossed with leaf shapes; it was the kind of speciality biscuit tin the supermarkets liked to bring out at Christmas, and I could see straight away why a child would think it special. Harry opened the lid and quickly showed us the contents which, as he'd said, were essentially a random pile of stones. 'Mustn't touch, of course,' he said, closing the lid again carefully. 'There'll be some very important order in this seemingly random pile, and if it's disturbed he will not be happy ...'

I nodded, thinking of Kieron and how nobody messed with his various childhood collections. That one I completely understood.

'Oh, and as I was just explaining to Mike,' Harry added, 'we still need to cover food. About which he's particularly pernickety.'

I grabbed my pen once more. 'No juice,' I said, as I began to write it down.

'And that's just the tip of the iceberg,' Harry commented. 'At the moment – and this has been the case for about a year now – I'm afraid Georgie will only eat white food.'

'*Really?*' Both my and Mike's eyebrows made a bolt for the ceiling. And remained aloft as Harry nodded his confirmation. 'Afraid so.'

'What, as in *all* white?' Mike asked. I could almost see his brain whirring.

'As in rice?' I said. 'That's the only white food I can think of.' I noticed my voice had become something of a plaintive squeak. How on earth would I cater for *that*?

'It's not quite that extreme,' Harry reassured us. 'He calls it "white" but perhaps a more correct word is "light". He is keen on "light" generally. And where food's concerned that means things like pasta in cheese sauce, for example. Most cereals, cheese on toast, macaroni cheese ... actually, I've said that already, haven't I? Don't look so alarmed,' he said, chuckling. 'Cook's put a list of "safe" foods in the folder for you, and, honestly, it's not as short as you might imagine. And he gets by at school, so there must be a reasonable amount of regular stuff on there ...'

Oh, dear God, I thought. *This just gets better and better.* And just to prove me right, Jenson chose that moment to make his second appearance.

'Am I okay to come down now?' he asked from the doorway. 'I wasn't taking the piss earlier, honest. Where's Georgie anyway? You want me to show him his new room?'

Great, I thought, conscious of Harry sitting with us. Making such a wonderful impression. 'Language, lad,' Mike checked him. 'You know the rules well enough. But, yes, that's a good idea. Let's all take him up, shall we?'

So that's what we did, trooping single file up the stairs with Jenson, as the official 'room shower', taking the lead. And for reasons of his own, it seemed – reasons for which we should perhaps have been prepared. 'Ta da!' he announced, swinging the bedroom door open. 'Georgie gets the girly room!'

I glared at him and pulled him away from the doorway. 'Stop being silly, Jenson. And don't worry, Georgie,' I added, making space so he could see it himself. 'It's only for a few days, love – after that you'll be in a different room, okay?'

Though I hadn't actually stipulated how *many* days – that would, of course, depend on what was going to happen with Jenson – it seemed even a few minutes were going to prove too much, because Georgie looked as if he was facing the jaws of death. Then, without warning, he let out a scream that was so ear-splitting that I actually clamped my hands over my ears.

Harry was quick to try and console him – though again, I noticed, this involved no physical contact. 'Shh, lad,' he soothed. 'It's okay, it's okay, it's okay … Casey didn't know, you see. That's all. She didn't know. It's okay …'

But Georgie carried on screaming, until, abruptly, he spoke. 'Imagine what you all look like to them,' he said, staccato-style. 'All pink and yellow. Episode 2. Imagine. All pink and yellow.'

Mike and I exchanged helpless bewildered looks as this continued, then it finally hit me – how dozy was I? – that I should shut the bedroom door. And once I did so the screaming and rambling stopped instantly, though I noticed Georgie was now physically shaking.

'My fault,' Harry said. 'I'm so sorry – completely slipped my mind, that. It's pink. Georgie hates pink – pink and anything pinkie-red, as well, to be exact about it. What a thing for me to forget.' He looked sheepishly at me. 'I don't suppose you have another room free, do you?'

This was beginning to feel surreal, and now everyone seemed to be looking in my direction, as if I could magically snap my fingers and whistle one up. Jenson, in particular, had a distinct 'I hope you're not thinking what I think you might be thinking' face on. But he needn't have worried. Though Georgie's needs were many and very evident, there was no way I'd add to Jenson's more subtle woes by evicting him, however much he'd wound the other boy up.

And, of course, I did have another room. Not ideal, of course, but functional. I nodded at Harry. 'How is he with double beds and beige?'

Not entirely happy, it seemed, even if this time we were spared what I assumed was a taste of what constituted a 'freak-out'. Two of the walls were beige, but the other two Mike had papered – a coffee-coloured background, with subtle chocolate and mocha coloured flowers. Which I'd chosen myself, in the January sales, and which had seemed a good idea at the time.

Time for a rethink, perhaps. 'It's the contrast,' Harry explained, as Georgie muttered disconsolately beside him. 'The wallpapered walls, I think. He's used to his room being quite bland – all one colour. Though we might be able to talk him round,' he suggested hopefully. 'Given a little time, anyway.'

I wondered what time he generally finished his working day. It was gone six already. I was also aware of how, judging from his doubtful expression, 'might' was the operative word.

Mike could obviously see that as well. 'No worries,' he said brightly. 'Jenson, lad, go and get your trainers on. You and I can nip down to B&Q and grab a pot of emulsion. Sixty-minute makeover time!' He chuckled and grinned at Georgie. 'How does that sound?'

How does that sound? I thought. *Like bang goes my flipping wallpaper …*

Chapter 11

True to Mike's promise, and with some enthusiastic assistance from Jenson, the spare room was made over in no time. And though there was still a whiff of emulsion lingering in the air when we got up there, Georgie seemed happy enough – having purposefully walked in and inspected it – to cast his eyes around without becoming agitated.

Indeed, once we'd taken all his belongings up, he seemed keen to go to bed. 'Georgie is yawning,' he announced, as soon as we'd trooped back down to the kitchen and seen Harry off. 'I go to bed at seven o'clock sharp.'

He then turned around – before I'd barely even had time to answer – and walked out of the kitchen and straight up the stairs.

Jenson, who was busy rinsing out a paint roller for Mike, sniggered. 'He's so –'

'Jenson!' I admonished, following Georgie out of the kitchen.

'Come on, lad,' chivvied Mike. 'We made a deal about telly, didn't we? And if you don't get that done you'll miss the start of your programme, won't you?'

Meanwhile, I followed Georgie up the stairs. Except when I got to the landing, it was to find that he wasn't in the bedroom, but instead standing patiently outside the closed bathroom door.

Unsure what he was doing, or, indeed, what he expected of me, I opened it – perhaps he needed the loo or something – but at the same time I pointed to the bedroom. 'All your things are in there, ready,' I said. 'And I've emptied out some drawers ready for you as well. You can transfer all your clothes into them now, if you like. And your pyjamas and toothbrush will be in your suitcase as well, won't they? I'm happy to help if you want me to.'

Georgie smiled – the first proper smile I'd seen from him so far, which lit his face up – and, looping a hank of his curtain of blond hair over his ear, trotted into the room and clicked open his case.

Unsure whether to start helping, and deciding against it for the moment, I stood in the doorway while he delved for his night things and wash bag.

He then stood up and having told me 'Georgie is yawning. Tomorrow', headed back across the landing to the bathroom. This time he went in and shut the door.

I decided to wait for him, and after a couple of minutes he emerged, in his pyjamas, holding his neatly folded school uniform under his arm. He'd also washed his face, I could see – the hair around his temples was damp and clinging – and I reflected that, for all the challenges I might have with this little boy, personal hygiene was unlikely to be one of them. Which would be refreshing, in more ways than one.

This time, however, it was as if he couldn't see me, because he made no eye contact or acknowledgement as he went back into his bedroom and carefully laid down his school clothes. Then, the job done, he simply walked up to the bedroom door and, once again without acknowledgement, shut the door.

'All settled, then?' asked Mike, looking up from the TV, when I went back downstairs.

'I presume so,' I said, shrugging. 'He's gone into his room and shut the door, so I assume he wants to sleep.'

'What a baby!' observed Jenson, with a disparaging look on his face. 'Who goes to bed at seven o'clock?'

'Erm, you, young man, if you carry on with that attitude,' said Mike mildly. 'Georgie's our guest, just like you are, so we'll have less of that, okay?'

Jenson grunted, but I was pleased to see an expression of slight contrition. Mike didn't need to raise his voice with him, I was beginning to notice. He seemed to have a natural authority with him. His height? Mike was a big man, and I sensed Jenson responded to that. I wondered if he'd ever known his own father.

I left them to it and went into the kitchen to start on supper. For all that he was wrong to take the mickey, Jenson

116

was right. It did seem early for a 9-year-old. But perhaps that was what worked for him, given that he'd always lived in a children's home – they could be hectic places, especially at those times, so perhaps it was less stressful for him to go to his room.

I also remembered that I'd read that children on the autism spectrum were often exhausted, because they expended so much mental energy trying to make sense of an environment that was so alien to them. It was also strange, I thought, how he referred to himself in both the first and the third person.

I rummaged in the veg rack and pulled out some potatoes, noticing the paint roller still dripping watery beige emulsion into the sink after its unexpected deployment. Still, I thought, at least he settled quickly again after that episode. Perhaps the 'freak-outs' wouldn't be quite as worrying as I'd first thought.

Though I wouldn't be counting chickens. Not just yet.

Mike was already washed and dressed before I was out of bed the next morning. I was awake – well, sort of – but when he came back up and popped his head around the bedroom door I was sneaking a few extra minutes.

'Cup of coffee, love,' he said. 'But you might want to get up anyway.' His voice was low and he was cocking his head slightly as he put the mug down on my bedside table. 'Young Georgie's standing on the landing holding his toothbrush,' he added.

I abandoned my sneaky five minutes and rubbed the sleep from my eyes. 'Standing?'

'Just standing there. Toothbrush and uniform in hand. I said good morning, but he seemed too preoccupied to hear me.'

'Preoccupied with what?'

'Preoccupied with staring at the bathroom door, I presume.'

I threw the duvet off. 'Go on, love,' I said. 'You go down and start your breakfast. I'll deal with it. Probably just waiting for Jenson to come out or something.'

Except he wasn't. Because, once I'd wriggled into my school run top and leggings, I put a head round Jenson's bedroom door to check.

I pulled it to again – Jenson could have an extra ten minutes yet – then knelt down to where Georgie was still standing, looking impassively at the centre of the door. I pushed it open, and then knelt down beside him.

'Morning, lovely!' I said brightly, just about checking my natural urge to make physical contact by ruffling his hair or giving his hand a friendly squeeze. He turned his gaze to mine. It was obviously a better option to be more on his level, I decided. Less threatening, perhaps.

He looked at me, then back to the door, and then he raised his finger and pointed. 'No Georgie,' he said. 'No Georgie on there. No Jenson.'

I stood up again, and tried to usher him into the bathroom using gestures. 'Yes, Georgie,' I said. 'It's Georgie's bathroom too, now. It's everyone's bathroom. Jenson's, and me and Mike's. And now Georgie's as well. We can all use it whenever we like, see?'

It took him a moment to process this, and then he stepped into the room. He still looked slightly doubtful for a second, then, once again, he turned around and closed the door in my face.

I smiled to myself, deciding to call the contact from the children's home, Sylvia something. Perhaps I needed more info on his usual morning rituals.

I also peeked into his room before heading back downstairs, and was intrigued to see he'd laid out a line of his special stones on the carpet. It was a row of ten, precisely placed about six inches from the door threshold. And precise in choice as well; I knew from having had a chance to see the collection that he had stones in a variety of shapes and colours. But these were all of a similar kind, which presumably held some significance. I stared at them for some seconds. *Nope. Not a clue!* There was no way, I decided, as I went to join Mike in the kitchen, that I could fathom what went on in this kid's mind.

Most cereals, as Harry had told us, were listed on Georgie's 'safe' list, so he and Jenson could both have Rice Krispies today.

'And what about a packed lunch?' Mike asked, as he poured himself a second coffee.

I shook my head. 'No need. He has school dinners, apparently. I don't know how they manage it, but I'm mighty glad they do. That's one change that would stress me just as much as it would Georgie.'

'Georgie what?' asked a voice. We both turned around to see Jenson, ready for school, in the way that meant 'ready' in Jenson-land anyway, i.e. tousled and looking like he'd slept in his uniform – a talent he seemed to have in spades.

'Georgie nothing,' I said, keen to steer the conversation elsewhere. 'Come on, sit down and have some cereal and then I'll sort out your hair.'

Mike, getting up now, gave Jenson's unruly mop a quick ruffle. 'Don't listen to Casey,' he laughed. 'Your hair's just fine, mate. But you be a good boy for her, okay? She's got two of you to think about now, and I don't want to be getting home and hearing either of you've played her up, okay?'

Jenson nodded. But then he grimaced, having clearly thought of something. 'I don't have to walk into school with him, do I?'

Mike laughed again. 'I can't see that, mate, can you? You'll be off like a whippet soon as the car door is opened, won't you? No, of course you don't have to. That's fine.'

I threw Mike a look. *So much for nurturing relationships, then!* I thought. There was me, trying to encourage bridge-building between them, and here was my husband happily widening the divide!

'What's wrong with them walking into school together?' I asked him.

'There's nothing wrong with it, love,' Mike said mildly. 'I'm just saying that not all kids want to walk into school together, that's all. Siblings, particularly,' he added. 'Even if they get on brilliantly at home.'

And, of course, in his quiet way, he was making an important point. Because I recalled that Riley and Kieron would probably have walked over broken glass rather than have to walk into school together. And they had their own sets of friends, just as Jenson and Georgie had. No, Mike was right. I shouldn't push things artificially. 'You're right, love,' I conceded. 'Jenson, that's fine. You can run ahead to catch your friends up. I'm going to be taking Georgie into his classroom in any case.'

At which point, the boy himself appeared, looking, despite the incongruous flowing blond locks, as neat and tidy as Jenson looked dishevelled.

And Georgie seemed to do everything with the same attention to detail. As Mike headed off – something to which Georgie seemed oblivious – he pulled his chair out carefully, sat down on it without ceremony, and sat silently, hands in lap, while I poured cereal into his bowl.

'Krispies are good,' he said, finally.

'Yes, they are,' I agreed, conscious of the need to try and forewarn him of what was happening. 'And once you've eaten them it will almost be time to go to school. And we're going in my car, do you remember? Like Harry told you?'

Georgie nodded. 'My new family. Different car.'

'Yeah,' Jenson interjected. 'Cos you ain't got no family, do you?' But before I could speak, Georgie provided his own retort.

'Liz told the Brigadier that the Doctor was all alone in the world. He had no family on this earth.'

Which effectively silenced Jenson, but also surprised me. I knew it was just some random line out of *Doctor Who*, but it seemed so profound, so clearly linked to what Jenson had said to him, that despite my knowing it was probably just a case of certain words triggering certain utterances, it made me feel so sad for him. For both boys. Because it seemed to have struck a chord with Jenson, as well. Looking suddenly sad himself, he scraped his chair back and left the room, while Georgie sat oblivious, happily chomping on his cereal.

Dropping the boys at school went without incident, but after introducing myself to Rowena, Georgie's learning-support assistant, I found my contemplative – and inexplicably rather morose – mood was still with me by the time I reached home.

Perhaps it was just the unusual way in which Georgie interacted with the world that triggered it, but I felt this real sense of sadness that there was a need for people like me and Mike – that there were so many pint-sized lost souls in the world, having to navigate their way through life as best they could.

I decided to hold off on the housework for a little while, and instead to phone Sylvia, the (presumably now redeployed) manager of Georgie's children's home. And she was as brisk and warm and jolly as I'd expected, with the sort of lilt to her voice that cheered you up just by listening.

I didn't know whether it was something she'd cultivated as a result of years of having to patiently manage the lives of children like Georgie, or just a gift, but either way it was like a balm on my grumpy mood.

'Ah, that'll be because there were no photos,' she cheerfully explained, after I'd told her about Georgie waiting by the bathroom door and us not having the slightest idea why. Not to mention how to shift him without touching him and upsetting him. 'So the solution is really easy,' she went on. 'He will have been confused about whether it was his bathroom or not. We had four of them at the home, and with so many children it just made life easier if they were all allocated specific ones to use. Hence the pictures. We had photos and names sellotaped on each one, so Georgie would have been looking for a door with his.'

'What a brilliant idea,' I said. 'I can easily do that. Any other helpful snippets? I'm obviously anxious to help him settle as soon as possible.'

And equally predictably, Sylvia had several. 'Well, images are the main thing, so if you can festoon your home with lots of them, you'll find day-to-day life with Georgie runs much more smoothly. Pinning pictures of shoes on the front of shoe cupboards, coats on the front of coat cupboards – that sort of thing is really helpful for him. Another thing you might like to do, since you're at it, is to be a bit creative and draw three big clocks.'

'Clocks? We have several in the house already. You mean as well as this?'

'Yes,' she said. 'So you can make them representative. One for breakfast time, lunchtime and dinnertime. And, again, use pictures. On the breakfast one, for example, you might want to stick on pictures of what he likes to have for breakfast, a plate of toast, say, or a bowl of porridge – you see?'

I did see. What a simple and brilliant idea!

'And in terms of how much of this sort of thing you do, the sky's the limit, really,' Sylvia finished. 'Really depends how you feel about having your home decked out like a reception class classroom. But all these little things – right down to a picture of a glass of milk on the fridge … anything that aids communication is a bonus. What people tend to underestimate is just how hard a boy like Georgie finds it to do something as simple as get across that he's thirsty. This way, he can simply point. So much less stressful for him.'

Sylvia made it all sound so simple and so obvious. I suddenly remembered a couple of children I had worked with at school. Both on the autism spectrum, they had carried around picture boards, and their teachers would change the pictures each day to correspond with whatever lessons they had. If they had Chemistry, for example, there would be a picture of a Bunsen burner, and if they had biology, a picture of the parts of a flower.

'But one warning,' Sylvia finished, after her 'can-do' list of positives. 'Georgie doesn't seem to feel pain like other children, so be sure to watch out for him hurting himself.'

'Doesn't he physically feel it?' This was difficult to imagine.

'Well, let's just say that he doesn't seem to articulate feeling it. He can go off like a bottle of pop if he feels emotionally unsettled, but where physical hurt's concerned he's a bit of an enigma. I have no idea about the physiology of such a thing, obviously, but this is not a child who is going to burst into tears if he cuts his knee.'

She went on to recount that a couple of years back, when Georgie had thrown himself at a wall in his frustration, he had broken his arm. 'But the only reason we knew,' she said, 'was because we got it X-rayed, hours later. And that was only because someone noticed he was holding it slightly strangely. Not a whimper of pain. It was incredible. None at all.'

It was a sobering piece of information to file away, that, and, as I put the phone down, I reflected that I'd learned more about the specifics of Georgie's autism in that one twenty-minute phone call than I had in several hours of research. It was a reminder that every child is an individual, with specific needs and tendencies – autistic children included.

I was also grateful to have Sylvia on tap. What had come across strongly was how much she cared, endorsed further by her instruction to call her any time – day or night – if I had questions or anxieties or a crisis.

That done, I spent a happy morning, courtesy of the previous season's Argos catalogue and the internet, cutting and sticking all sorts of images for around the house. And an even happier afternoon, with Riley, having remembered she had a laminator, creating wipeable, splash-resistant cards for almost everything, from the mug cupboard to the bathroom cabinet to the DVD drawer beneath the telly, all of which I'd have the boys help me put up once I'd collected them from school.

But I should have expected that there might be a fly stuck in my ointment. My mobile rang just as I was climbing into my car to do the pick-up. It was Marie Bateman, with sobering news.

'I know it's eleventh hour,' she said, 'but I've literally just come out of the meeting. Jenson's contact visit tomorrow has been cancelled.'

'Why?' I spluttered, already imagining the upset this would cause poor Jenson, and – as a consequence – the calm environment of our home.

'The boyfriend, Gary – sorry, fiancé – has moved in with Karen, basically.'

'And?' I asked, knowing that there would be slightly more to it. You didn't cancel contact without good reason. Oh, poor Jenson.

'Because there are question marks over him,' Marie said. 'Bit of a bad boy. No need to go into details, but he's had something of a chequered past. Not involving kids, as far as I know, but he still needs to be police-checked. You know how these things work.'

Indeed I did. 'But couldn't Karen see Jenson elsewhere, like they did last time?'

'Yes, in theory. And that was what was planned. Except she's being so antagonistic there's a concern that there's more to this. We think that it's Gary's influence, but Karen is actually saying that if her Gary can't go to the contact then she won't either. Hence the decision. Which I know is going to upset Jenson dreadfully, but I'm hoping we'll be able to reschedule it for early next week. Sorry,' she said again, after a short pause. 'I'm all too aware that it's you who's going to have to deal with the fall-out.'

And attendant freak-out, no doubt, I thought. Wonderful.

Chapter 12

I was dreading breaking the news to Jenson. He was so looking forward to seeing his mum, and I couldn't help cursing her for being so heartless. Unbelievable that she would rather score points against social services than make her poor child feel loved and wanted. I was also concerned about the implications of what she'd done. She was his mum, for God's sake – didn't she want to *see* him?

I decided not to break the news straight after school, but after tea. In my experience hungry kids were much more easily wound up than kids with full stomachs.

'Hope you're both hungry, guys!' I said brightly, as we pulled out from the school drive. 'Lovely fish, mashed potatoes and parsley sauce for tea!'

Parsley sauce, that was, with very, very tiny flecks of parsley. I glanced through the rear-view mirror and noted the small contented smile on Georgie's face. He was looking down at his cupped hands again, in that intense way he had, as if seeing them for the very first time. I wasn't even sure if he was listening, but no matter, Jenson was. 'No mushy peas?' he said. 'You got to have mushy peas if it's fish – it's the rule.'

'Mushy peas for all the rest of us, love, don't worry. But not for Georgie. I don't think he likes them, do you, Georgie?'

Jenson turned to Georgie. 'Is it cos they're all bogie coloured, Georgie? Bogie green. Mmm. Yummy yummy. Lovely and *greeeeen*.'

'Jenson, knock it off please,' I said. 'Stop being silly. You –'

'Giant maggots!' Georgie suddenly exclaimed. 'With green slime, unleashed by BOSS – Biomorphic Organisational Systems Supervisor. It killed the miner.' He paused and turned his head. 'Green death.'

Through the mirror I could see Jenson's jaw drop. Georgie, nonplussed, went back to studying his hands, while his small tormentor decided he'd perhaps leave off the tormenting and look out of the window instead.

I smiled to myself. There were definitely some plus-points to kids being afraid of things they didn't under-stand. And as a defence against being teased, it was priceless.

Once we got home, Georgie noticed the results of my day's labours straight away, and walked slowly around each room, studying every picture carefully. His eyes positively lit up when he saw the clocks I'd created, with their times and what each one represented. He turned and grinned at me, even making eye contact very fleetingly.

'This is good,' he said. 'Good, Casey. This is Georgie's house.'

I felt my throat constrict a little, knowing what I knew and he didn't; that this was only to be his home temporarily. That, in all probability, just as he had settled in, they would find a permanent home for him, which would mean going through the whole trauma of moving once again. And not for the first time – since that was the nature of my work – I felt bad about it; something of a fraud.

I smiled anyway. 'Yes, it sure is, kiddo. And now you know where everything lives, you can help me look after you better, can't you?'

Luckily, Jenson wasn't around to hear that exchange, having gone straight up to his room to change out of his uniform. I had a feeling he already felt a bit pushed out by Georgie, as would any child who felt they'd been usurped by a new arrival, which was why child-care books made so much of all the things you had to do when bringing home a new baby.

I also had a hunch he resented the fact that Georgie was staying for considerably longer than he was. Mad, when you thought how desperate he was to get back home again, but then, human emotions weren't always logical.

I had decided to eat with the boys, rather than waiting for Mike and eating later, as I felt my presence around the table, sharing a family meal, would be important – leading by example, as it were. And as I took their meals and tumblers of milk through to the dining room I was pleased to find the atmosphere was actually one of conviviality. Yes, Jenson was making a big fuss about his upcoming mushy peas, to torment Georgie – licking his lips and waving his fork around, and generally being a bit silly – but, at that level, particularly since Georgie seemed to be ignoring it, I decided it might be best to ignore it myself.

Besides, I had something of my own to bring up, and though I wavered – should I take Jenson off to his room after we'd eaten? – I had a gut instinct that it might make the whole thing seem less portentous if I didn't make too big a deal of it. Present it as a logistical problem more than anything; perhaps that way he wouldn't read too much into it.

And it looked like I'd have an opportunity. Georgie, his glass empty, started pointing to it and looking at me. He obviously wanted another drink.

'Do me a favour, love,' I said to Jenson, since he had already finished eating. 'Come into the kitchen and help me with dessert, yes? And a drink for Georgie,' I added. 'There's a love. Oh, by the way,' I said lightly, once we were safely out of earshot. 'I know it's going to disappoint you, love, but unfortunately your visit to see your mum tomorrow's had to be postponed. They're going to rearrange it for as soon as possible, obviously – just not tomorrow. I'm so sorry, sweetheart,' I finished, handing him the fresh tumbler of milk.

I watched Jenson's face set into a rigid angry mask. 'They can't do that!' he said. 'Who said so anyway? Is it the social or her who've done the cancelling?'

'Your social worker, love,' I said carefully. 'Marie did.' There was no need to tell him the real truth about it. Indeed, I sincerely hoped he wouldn't have to find out. 'I'm sorry,' I said again. 'I know she'll rearrange it just as soon as she possibly can.'

'Why, though?' he persisted, as I rummaged in the fridge for yoghurts. 'Has someone said owt about me? I bet they have. I bet you anything it was that bloody old –'

'*Jenson*,' I said calmly. 'I promise you, it's not that. This has absolutely nothing to do with anything you have done or not done. This is just stuff that the grown-ups have to sort out. You've done nothing wrong,' I repeated. 'Nothing wrong at *all*. And I'm sure Marie will get back to us just as soon as she can, and in the meantime, perhaps –'

'Fuck off!' Jenson said, immediately slamming down the glass. He banged it down with such force that milk slopped over the worktop, but thankfully I'd chosen sensibly – it was plastic. 'Fuck *off*!' He was by now on his way back through to the dining room. 'And *you* can fuck off as well!' he railed, pointing at a startled Georgie. 'You can specially fuck off, you fucking retard!'

'Jenson!' I said firmly. 'This isn't helping anything. Now would you please sit back down and calm down and finish your tea. I know you're upset, but I won't have you talking like that in this house, you hear me?'

But Jenson was too enraged now for my words to have any impact. 'Fuck *off*!' he yelled again, running to the dining room door. 'And yeah, I *do* hear, okay? Just like I hear everything you say to him!' He glared at Georgie again. 'All your stupid pictures. Fucking retard! You can shove the fucking lot of them up your arse!'

Jenson thundered up the stairs, leaving both Georgie and me staring. But then I realised that Georgie wasn't just staring; he'd begun rocking. He'd clamped his hands to his ears and was rhythmically rocking; back and forth, back and forth, his eyes fixed on the middle distance, his expression glassy eyed and weird and pained.

I went across to him, anxious not to startle him with sudden movements.

'It's okay, sweetheart,' I said softly. 'Jenson was just a bit upset. He's just angry because he's not having a very good day.'

I was close to Georgie now, and was just dithering about whether or not to touch him when, quite without warning, he emitted a high-pitched scream. It was so piercing and so loud that it made me take a step back involuntarily. Which was just as well, because he clearly didn't want me anywhere near him. But as I backed away the intensity of the scream got even stronger. *Now what the hell did I do?*

It might have been a few seconds, but it might equally have been minutes, but I was still standing there dithering, trying to decide upon a course of action, when salvation appeared to me in the form of Mike, who had just got home from work.

'What the – ?' he began, till I flapped a hand to silence him and could bundle him back into the hall.

'I don't know what to *do!*' I whispered helplessly, glancing back at where Georgie, his blond locks swinging back and forth along with him, continued to scream the place down. 'Jenson kicked off,' I hissed, by way of explanation, 'which is what seems to have started it. And I don't know what on earth to do to try and stop it!'

Mike looked past me, back into the kitchen, where Georgie continued screaming. If it went on much longer he would surely lose his voice. Yet I was heedful of Harry's warning about how carefully I needed to deal with him. Mike, though, was obviously in a more bullish frame of mind. 'Georgie?' he barked, in his most deep and authoritarian tone. 'It's okay, mate. No one is angry any more now. There's nothing to be scared of. Calm down. It's okay.'

The decibel level suddenly subsided markedly, I noticed, which seemed a good thing. Perhaps it meant he was listening. He clearly responded well to the depth of Mike's voice.

'It's okay now,' Mike said again, keeping a prudent two or three feet from him. 'There is nothing to be scared of now. Everything's okay.'

The screaming, bit by bit, began to morph into a whimper, and though Georgie still rocked and still had his hands clamped over his ears there was a sense that the tsunami of distress was now passing. He was finally beginning to calm down.

But it was a fragile sort of calm; he still seemed wired and not quite with us, a situation not improved by the reappearance of Jenson, who had obviously been upstairs sobbing, while he tackled his own demons. His face was wet and streaked and filthy. And seeing the three of us, he promptly burst into tears all over again. 'I'm sorry,' he sobbed. 'I'm sorry, Casey.' He gulped a little, wiped his eyes and turned his gaze to Georgie. 'An' I'm sorry to you as well,' he sniffed, marching across to Georgie, where, with a wobbly little smile, he apologised again.

What happened next seemed to happen in slow motion, as is often the case when something comes at you right out of the blue. Georgie removed his hands from his ears and, with a grimace, accompanied by an inhuman-sounding growl, leapt from his chair and literally launched himself at Jenson. And it was some launch, as well; he pretty much hurled himself at him, as if unexpectedly called upon to wrestle a hungry bear. You couldn't have witnessed a more dramatic, full-on, fists-flying assault if you'd been watching a Tom and Jerry cartoon.

Except this wasn't funny, this was ugly, proper violence. This might have only been two 9-year-old boys having a scrap, except that Georgie clearly wasn't like most 9-year-old boys. I'd read about it, heard about it, taken it all in – but that was nothing compared to seeing it in action. And something else was clear: Georgie might not be able to feel pain that deeply, but he sure as hell was good at inflicting it.

'Arrgh!' screamed Jenson, easily matching Georgie's earlier volume. 'Mike, gerr 'im off me!' he said, as dining chairs clattered to the floor around them. 'Gerr 'im *off* me! He's a fucking nutter!'

It was probably only a matter of moments before Mike managed to do so, but it was a much bigger job that I think even he expected, and once they'd been separated I was horrified to see what damage had already been done. There was a nasty graze beginning to swell on Jenson's cheek and, clutched tightly in Georgie's fist, a shockingly big clump of Jenson's hair.

And, of course, Jenson – now livid – was anxious to return the compliment, and had begun trying to thrash around and wriggle from Mike's grip. 'Lemme go!' he screeched. 'I'm going to fucking kill him, I am. *Kill* him!'

'No, you're *not*,' Mike said firmly. 'You are both going to *calm down*.'

Which Georgie by now *had* already done, after a fashion. Seemingly spent from his turn as a Tasmanian devil, once Mike had managed to extricate Jenson from his clutches he'd simply flopped. Flopped against *me*, more specifically. Though 'flopped' wasn't really the word. He now leaned against me in the same way a step-ladder would: completely rigid, with his feet planted squarely on the floor, and with his head – he had his back to me, and I held his upper arms loosely – a heavy blond weight against my chest.

Jenson was still struggling, but with slightly less conviction now. 'Just lemme go to my room,' he sobbed to Mike now. 'Just let me get *out* of here, *please*.'

Mike slowly released his grip. I could see he was still ready for further action, but we could soon tell Jenson had no fight left in him. Clutching his head – which, poor lad, must have been stinging like fury – he turned and once again thundered back off up the stairs.

I waited for the inevitable door slam, and he obliged me. Then I turned to Mike, my rigid human shield still leant against me.

'Well,' I mouthed helplessly. 'What now?'

In the end, by a combination of cajoling and gently nudging, I managed to 'herd' a now completely mute Georgie into the living room. He was still glassy-eyed, but when I said the word '*Countdown*' he seemed to shift gear, and seemed happy enough to let me arrange him on the sofa and wait meekly for the remote while I switched on the TV. Thank heavens for Sky, I thought, scrolling through the planner. Not to mention my great foresight in series linking the programme.

I returned to the kitchen to find Mike filling the kettle.

'Well, that was fun,' I said, bringing the dirty dishes to the sink. I felt so sorry for my poor husband – what a thing to come home to after a hard day at work! 'God knows how we bring them back from this,' I said, sighing. That bald patch of Jenson's would be something to see. 'God, I hope this sort of thing isn't going to become a regular occurrence!'

Mike shook his head as he spooned instant coffee into mugs for us. 'I sincerely hope not,' he said. 'And nothing to do with poor Jenson himself, obviously, but perhaps it's for the best that he's off pretty soon, eh? I have a hunch that having the two of them here isn't going to work.'

I nodded. 'I suspect you're right. But there's been a development on that score.' I told him about the contact visit cancellation. *And* the reason.

'Oh, dear,' he said. 'That sounds a bit ominous, love, doesn't it?'

I agreed that it did. It was echoing my very thoughts. 'But let's not jump to conclusions, eh, love? How about your dinner? Shall I finish clearing this lot away and warm yours up?'

'I'm not sure I fancy anything just now, after all that.' He grinned ruefully. 'I can always microwave it later – if and when I get my appetite back.'

I found a smile and dredged it up while Mike poured hot water onto our coffees. 'Well, there's a positive, at least,' I said. 'Because mine's disappeared as well. So at this rate, by the time one of them goes elsewhere we'll have both lost a couple of pounds, won't we?'

We both laughed because, as everyone knows, laughter's the best medicine. But violence is always shocking, no matter how young the pugilists, and, duly shocked, I only had one thought in my head – that I might soon be tearing my own hair out.

Chapter 13

'What colour is a rainbow, Casey?'

Not the first thing you expect to be asked in the morning, particularly the very second you open your bedroom door. Nevertheless, that was what Georgie obviously badly needed to know. He was standing right outside it – literally, nose to wood with it. I almost jumped out of my skin.

'Oh, you gave me a fright, Georgie!' I said, clutching my chest for effect as I mentally tried to remember the rhyme. *Richard of York Gave Battle in Vain*, that was it. But before I could recite the colours, Georgie had another question. 'What colour is a chameleon if it goes into a rainbow?' Then, bizarrely, 'Do the Aztecs eat meat?'

This was new, I decided, as I tried to come up with answers, but then I realised that Georgie didn't even seem to want them. I could tell as I spoke that he wasn't listening, and was back locked in his own train of thought. Perhaps thinking up questions was just a stress-relieving strategy – and after last night there was certainly plenty of that fizzing about.

'I tell you what,' I finished. 'How about you go downstairs ready for your breakfast, eh? I'll just use the bathroom and then I'll be there.'

Wincing slightly as I passed my own grinning mugshot on the bathroom door, I reflected that today might be a stressful one as well. Though both boys had settled again, after the aftermath of their fight – even sharing opposite ends of the same sofa to watch TV with us – I wasn't naïve enough to suppose they were now friends. For one thing, Georgie didn't 'do' friends, not in the way other kids did, and with a weeping bald patch to remind him what Georgie *could* do, I had no doubt that Jenson would be keen to get him back.

I followed Georgie down to find both boys sitting waiting patiently in the dining room, having chosen seats that gave them both a view of the telly in the living room, through the French doors.

'Morning, all!' I said brightly, picking up the Krispies for Georgie and pouring them into his bowl for him. That done, I went to do the same for Jenson.

'Can I have Coco Pops, instead?' he said.

'Can I *please* have Coco Pops, Jenson? And yes, of course you can. I'll go and fetch them.'

I knew why Jenson was doing this; it was to wind up poor Georgie. Having homed in on the white-food thing like an Exocet missile, he was obviously keen to target it at every opportunity. I would simply ignore it, though, because it seemed to me that Georgie didn't even notice. As long as he had what he wanted, it seemed he couldn't give a fig about what anyone else put in their mouths.

Not that Jenson wouldn't get this himself before long. At which point, I had no doubt that he would just try and find something else. The only question being what, and how soon.

'What we doing today, then?' Jenson asked me once I'd poured out his cereal. 'Seeing as how I won't be seeing my mum and Carley.' He seemed to think. 'That's unless Carley is seeing her. Is she? I bet she is.'

'No, love. Neither of you are – just like I told you yesterday. Anyway, Mike's had to pop into work for a couple of hours this morning, so we'll decide what to do with ourselves then, okay?'

Jenson frowned. 'Bet she's lying. She likes Carley way more than me. Bet they've decided to go girly shopping and just don't want me there.'

'Love, that's not the case, I promise you.'

'Bet it is.'

There was nothing I could say that would change his mind, clearly. Not without spelling out the real reason for the cancelled visit, which was the last thing I wanted to do. And perhaps he had good reason to think that might be the case. Perhaps that was something that happened often – how did I know? Once again I got this feeling that there was something more to their relationship; that, much as Jenson wanted to be wanted by his mother, there was this clear sense that he held a grudge against her.

Making myself a coffee, I thought back to what the neighbour had said about 'all that business with the little one'. It wasn't really anything to do with me – social services would obviously reach their own conclusions – but, given that they had flagged up some concerns regarding the fiancé, perhaps I should make it my business to find out.

Breakfast soon eaten and Mike due home from work imminently, I told the boys to go up and wash and dress. 'And while you're at it you can both tidy your bedrooms,' I said. 'Think you can do that?' I glanced at Georgie to see that he understood what I was saying. 'That sound good, Georgie? You know how to tidy your room, right?'

I ignored Jenson's snigger, and concentrated on Georgie, and was pleased to see that funny little smile cross his face. As he spent so much of his time looking so blankly at nothing, I decided it must have some significance. That he understood, perhaps? And that he felt comfortable with it? Just instinct, but then I would have to work on instinct. Till I got to know him better, that was all I had to go on. That and my experience with my own son.

If Georgie was anything like Kieron, of course, I would have nothing to worry about. Kieron would only operate in a room with complete order. Everything would have its own special place and he certainly wouldn't accept the thought of mess. And something told me that I was dealing with the same sort of mindset. Unlike most boys his age, but in the same way as Kieron, Georgie probably wouldn't dream of leaving dirty clothes on his floor or randomly

discarding toys and games. Children with such disposi-
tions, like Georgie – and also our last child, Abigail – did
have some perks, I decided.

The boys off upstairs, I went back into the kitchen to wash
the dishes. Annoyingly, it had started to pour down outside.
I switched on the radio and turned it up to drown the noise
out. If there was one thing I really hated, it was rain. I loved
the cold, I loved the heat, and I especially loved snow, but
rain just drained the cheer out of everything. Most annoyingly, it had that unique ability to scupper plans, and where
with snow you could simply make new, more exciting
plans, when it rained there was so much you couldn't do.

And I had had a plan: to take the boys to the woods. I
loved having a patch of woodland just yards from our front
door. Not only had it been one of the unexpected bonuses
of moving to our current house, it had also delighted us
with bluebells and wood anemones and primroses and, best
of all, since it had a proper babbling brook running through
it, with frogspawn and baby frogs as well.

And, naturally, it also had stones. But if it continued to
rain like this we'd have to schedule our visit for another day,
and I was just trying to think what else we could get up to
when I heard the front door go. Mike. Home from work.

'Hi, love! I'm back!' he called, as per usual, from the
hallway. I smiled as I put the kettle on for more coffee.

'It's awfully quiet in here,' he said, coming up behind me
to give me a hug. 'Come on, out with it, woman. What
have you done with them?'

'What, my little angels?' I laughed. 'Actually, they are both upstairs, cleaning. I am endeavouring to mould them in my image. By the way, what do you think we should do with them today? I did think it would be nice to take them to the woods and tire them out. But now it's raining.'

Mike peered out of the window. 'Not that hard. And it looks like it's easing up, too. So that sounds like a plan to me. But is there any chance of some boiled eggs and soldiers first?'

'You big baby,' I scolded, smacking him on the backside with the morning paper. 'Go on then. Long as you promise to be the one to take them down to the muddy bit by the stream. Do your David Bellamy bit while I stay on the grassy bit, because if I end up on my backside in the mud there will be hell to pay.'

'You big wuss,' he responded. Touché, then.

Even so, his breakfast made, I went upstairs and pulled clothes out for all weather eventualities, which was only sensible for summer outings in Britain: my very tatty combat pants, a lightweight baggy jumper that had seen better days and my not-at-all-fashionably-branded wellies. Very chic, I thought, taking my pyjamas off, ready to go and have a shower.

I'd just done so when the still air was once again disturbed by a high-pitched and now familiar scream. I stopped dead. It was obviously Georgie, and in distress.

Grabbing my combat pants and wriggling into them, then pulling a vest top over my head, I yanked the bedroom door open to find Georgie standing in the doorway to

Jenson's bedroom, still screaming and this time also point-ing. I then heard Jenson's voice from inside. 'Get lost, you freak!' he was yelling. 'Stop fucking screaming and sod *off*!'

Mike had by now joined us on the landing, and crossing it I could now see inside Jenson's bedroom. He was sitting on his bed looking cross.

Mike sidestepped Georgie, taking care not to touch him. 'What's going on, Jenson?' he said over the racket.

'Oh. My. God!' Jenson spluttered. 'What are you blam-ing *me* for? That freak just came in here and started scream-ing at me! I can't get no sense out of him. Look at him!'

'I'm not blaming you for anything,' Mike said calmly. 'I'm just asking you because Georgie is obviously too upset to speak.'

At the sound of his name, Georgie's screams got even louder. *God*, it occurred to me, *what are the neighbours thinking?*

Jenson crossed his arms over his chest and looked defi-antly back at Mike. 'I don't *know* what's wrong with him,' he said. 'How should I?'

'But why do you *think* he might be upset?' Mike persisted.

Jenson spread his palms now. 'I told you – I don't *know*!'

I knelt down close to Georgie. 'Love,' I said, 'I can see something's upset you, but you need to tell us what. Or show me. Otherwise we can't help you, can we?'

The screaming stopped as dramatically and instantly as it had started, and though I had absolutely no idea what had been the trigger in what I'd said I silently congratulated myself for having found a way through the din. Georgie then marched straight across the landing to his own bedroom, and pointed – very pointedly – at the line of stones just beyond his doorway.

I followed his eyes downwards – it was some kind of moat, I imagined, preventing entry. Had Jenson stepped over it? And then I remembered. I counted. There were nine stones. Before, there'd been ten.

'Did someone move a stone, Georgie?' I asked him, even though I already knew the answer.

Without saying a word, Georgie walked, shoulders down, to the bathroom door, where he pointed to the picture of Jenson.

'Did Jenson take your stone, sweetheart?'

'Jenson bad,' Georgie said. He then hung his head and returned to Jenson's doorway. Once there, he looked straight into the eyes of his tormentor, and promptly began screaming again.

'Jenson!' I called, above the noise. 'One of Georgie's stones is missing. He says you have it. Now will you please give it back to him. You obviously knew it would upset him, and if you don't want to be grounded I suggest you do as I ask right this minute.'

Mike, who was by now sitting on the bed with Jenson, patted his arm. 'Come on, lad, this isn't funny. Not when you do it to a boy like Georgie. It's just mean. You know that ...'

Jenson bridled. 'So's what he did to my fucking hair!'

'I know, lad, but two wrongs ...'

Jenson leapt up then. He reached under his pillow and produced the offending item, then, waving it around above his head for a moment, yelled 'Here it is, you fucking retard! You wan' it so bad? Well, you can have it!' With which he threw it, with unnerving accuracy, straight at Georgie's forehead.

Here we go again! I thought, as Georgie's hand flew to his temple and, meanwhile – it was obviously a lucky shot, after all – Jenson , looking mortified, tried to make a bolt for the door. Luckily, Mike grabbed him, and meanwhile (and quite forgetting about the various protocols) I grabbed Georgie and clamped my arms around him. Which again stopped him screaming, but now he started struggling instead, and, to my amazement, managed to shrug me off as easily as he would a coat. I didn't resist. He was obviously in some sort of shock, but it was only as he got free of me that I saw to what extent, because he immediately hurled himself across the room and slammed his whole body at the wall.

It happened so quickly but he must have done it three times in all – each time more violently than the last – before Mike could grab him from behind and wrestle him gently but firmly to the ground.

They stayed locked there, both rocking from side to side, for some minutes, Mike with his arms wrapped firmly round Georgie's torso, and with the boy's legs spread out in front, between his own. It almost looked like some horror-movie version of that dance – the one that goes 'Oops, upside your head', that people do at discos in long chains.

Jenson, as transfixed now as I was, hadn't moved, his bolt for freedom obviously having been forgotten. This was a whole other league of kids having freak-outs, I thought distractedly. I'd been in some scrapes with angry, self-loathing, behaviourally extreme children, but I'd never witnessed anything quite like this before – and certainly not in my own home. And nor had Jenson, I imagined. He had tears rolling down his cheeks again, and was shaking. He looked scared and appalled.

I followed his gaze. 'Look, Casey,' he said in a small voice. 'Look at his *head*.'

So I looked, and saw a fat thread of blood on Georgie's neck, which was running freely and beginning to soak into his hair. It wasn't from the stone; there was no sign that that had actually hurt him, and from where it seemed to come from my guess was a wound on the back of his head. Which wasn't surprising, given the animalistic way he'd thrown himself against the bedroom wall.

Another instinct kicked in. I mustn't alarm Georgie. Mustn't alarm either boy, in fact. Squeezing Jenson's hand to reassure him, I mouthed the word 'blood' to Mike. Forget the woods. We needed to get to A&E.

Chapter 14

Happily, despite the copious amount of blood, Georgie didn't need any stitches. 'It's typical of this sort of head wound,' the kindly and very patient A&E nurse explained. 'They bleed like anything, so they tend to look worse than they really are.' She grinned at Georgie, who had seemed in a daze since we'd got there. 'You're going to have to lose a clump of this gorgeous hair though!'

I half expected Jenson to whoop, or cry 'Touché!', or something similar, but, like all of us, he seemed to have had the stuffing knocked out of him, and merely stood there, looking on and looking miserable.

We made the journey home in silence, too, Georgie clutching his hank of bloody hair tightly to him. The nurse, though bemused by his insistence that she couldn't have it, had kindly popped it in a bag for him. And once home and I'd given both boys a glass of milk and a biscuit, we quickly put the day to bed as well. 'We start afresh tomorrow, okay, boys?' I told them as I led them both upstairs. 'Start over. Tomorrow is another day. In this house we don't carry things over till tomorrow, so we'll say no more on the matter, okay?'

'I can't believe all that just happened,' Mike said, once I was back downstairs. He patted the sofa, and I flopped down beside him. 'Just can't believe it,' he said again. 'D'you think having these two together is ever going to work?'

'I don't know, love,' I said honestly. 'But you know what? I'm too tired to even think about it properly. But you're right. Poor Georgie. It's like Jenson hates him. He's really made it his mission to go all out to torment the poor boy.'

'Steady on, love,' said Mike mildly. 'I don't think it's that bad. I think it's more that Jenson doesn't understand him. Which is different. And then naturally pushes buttons to see what'll happen next. Just usual kid stuff, if you ask me.'

I turned to face Mike, a little shocked. 'What, you mean like he just takes a healthy interest in the autism spectrum? Come *on*, love! You really don't think there's any malice in what Jenson does?'

Mike paused before answering, and I could tell he was choosing his words. And I felt annoyed. Was he siding with Jenson in all this? I was also, if I was honest, a little cross with myself. Like all the kids that came to us, Jenson had his issues, and displaying bad behaviours didn't mean he was a bad person. Just a troubled one. For which I knew I should make allowances. But, strangely, in this case, I was finding that hard to focus on. He seemed to have this unnerving ability to really wind me up.

'All I'm saying,' Mike continued, 'is that Georgie must be a puzzle to him – as I'm sure he is to any other kid of their age. Don't you remember when Kieron was little and how the other kids used to treat him? And how he never got invited to parties or anything? How all the other kids thought *he* was strange?'

'Of course I remember,' I said, back on the defensive. 'But they were never downright mean to him – I would never have stood for that!' I thought back. And in doing so, another thing occurred to me. 'And besides,' I said, 'Kieron didn't have *half* the problems Georgie has.'

I could see Mike's attention turning back to the TV, confirmed when he picked up the remote. And he was probably right. No point in discussing this while we were both so wound up. And bringing Kieron into the equation would only make me more volatile; I remembered very well how emotionally intense it had been, watching Kieron trying to navigate the business of relationships. Nothing in that department was ever straightforward for him. Some kids over-compensated by being over-protective, but the bulk of them – from nursery school onwards, pretty much – would simply see teasing him as sport; hiding a favourite pencil, or toy-of-the-moment, or knocking his carefully arranged towers of bricks down. And yes, maybe Mike was right – part of it was born out of curiosity. Wondering what might happen if they did X or Y. Perhaps Mike was right; I should try to be more patient with Jenson. But it was hard. Because I *could* see his malice.

* * *

Nevertheless, I tried, and though I was tested many times over the next few days I did make a concerted effort to educate Jenson, to try and help him understand Georgie a little more.

And I even told Kieron, though without getting the response I expected. 'Mum, he's 9!' he laughed. 'What else do you expect?'

I pulled a face. So he and his father – currently in the kitchen, preparing vegetables with Jenson – were both in cahoots on this, were they?

'So what do I do, then?' I bridled. 'Just let him get on with it? Just leave him to wind Georgie into such frenzy that he constantly screams the house down?'

'No, Mum,' Kieron said patiently. 'But you're expecting too much. You can't force friendships. You'll just make things worse. No one likes being told who they should and shouldn't like, and, once he decides, Jenson will either like Georgie or he won't. That's the way it works,' he said firmly, 'and there's nothing you can do about it.'

Typical Kieron, I thought. Bless him. Simplifying everything. It was all black and white to him – everything in between was just stuff that got in the way. And perhaps he had a point, I thought, looking across to Mike and Jenson busy in the kitchen while Georgie, gently rocking, was sitting watching TV. Perhaps I should stop trying to push them together and instead try to keep them more apart. Give them my time individually. Why on earth hadn't I thought of that before?

'Kieron,' I said, as I went to help with the dinner, 'you're a genius.'

'I am?' he asked, bemused. Then he regrouped. 'I mean, of course I am; I already knew that, Mum, obviously. But I *am*?'

'Yes, Mr Modest, you are.'

Armed with a new perspective, I had a new and different agenda, and began to make changes to our daily routine. With no date on the horizon for when Jenson's situation might be changing, I decided to work on the basis that he'd be with us for a few weeks yet, and that I should treat both the boys as if they were with us separately, and stop trying to treat them like siblings. And although this meant some extra work on my part, it soon started to pay dividends.

I began getting up half an hour early and waking up Georgie, so I could take him down and give him breakfast in peace and quiet. Then, with him fed and happily settled in front of the television, I would wake Jenson, bring him down and do likewise. During the school run I allowed Jenson to play on his DS, to keep him occupied, so there was no need to entertain himself baiting Georgie. And after school I'd let Georgie watch half an hour of *Doctor Who* while Jenson helped me prepare tea in the kitchen.

And by the Thursday of the following week I was feeling pretty pleased with myself. There had been hardly anything in the way of squabbles between the boys, and an atmosphere of calm mostly prevailed. I had even planned on going up to school with Riley and the little ones, as it was sports day and Jenson was running in one of the races, something about which he'd been really excited. But pride, as we all know, generally comes before a fall, and I was naturally about to be tripped up.

It was just after eleven – around playtime, I guessed – when my mobile began trilling inside my bag.

It was Andrea Cappleman. 'We'd like you to come and collect Jenson,' she told me.

'Why?' I asked her, already fearing the answer.

'Fighting,' she responded, exactly on cue.

'With Georgie?'

'With Georgie?' She sounded surprised. 'No, not as far as I know. I'm still not in possession of all the facts at this point, but there were three boys involved in this, one of whom was Jenson, and since it's sports day we've decided to exclude all of them, as a punishment –'

'Exclude them?' I asked, shocked.

'Yes, but only for the rest of the day. None will come clean about what happened – typical 9-year-olds – and since everyone seems determined to blame everyone else we've decided to send everyone home to reflect, in the hopes that they'll explain themselves tomorrow. Perhaps you'll have more luck – that's my hope, at least.'

I drove up to school feeling thoroughly cross. Georgie wasn't involved in sports day – it was the sort of unscheduled, noisy event that would only upset him, so it wasn't a worry that I'd miss anything he was doing. But I just felt this overwhelming irritation at Jenson. I understood perfectly that he had his demons to deal with, and the rational part of my mind acknowledged that acting out all the time was a natural result of this. But at the same time I felt exasperated that he'd already managed – by mid-morning – to completely sabotage his own day.

And I could tell by his expression when I arrived to collect him that missing sports day was on his mind as well. He scowled as I approached, but I could see he'd been crying, and when the school secretary opened the door for us to leave he didn't thank her.

'Jenson!' I chided. 'What do you say to Mrs Mason?'

But he was already marching off across the playground, seemingly deaf, leaving me frowning apologetically in his wake.

And he began with the usual 'it wasn't my fault' prattle immediately he got into the car.

'It never is!' I barked crossly, as I pushed the key into the ignition. 'It's always someone else's fault with you, isn't it, Jenson?'

'But it was!' he said, yanking the seatbelt across him. 'I told Miss Cappleman an' all, but did she listen? Did she hellus like!'

'So, tell me then,' I asked him. 'What happened? And no lies please.'

He stared resolutely out of the window as I pulled away from the kerb. 'Well?' I said. 'Are you going to tell me? Because it seems to me that all you've achieved so far today is to completely ruin your afternoon. Not to mention mine. None of which strikes me as very clever!'

He met my eyes through the rear-view mirror and his expression was one of fury. 'What's the fucking point?' he said. 'You're just like my fucking mum – you *all* are! Just take me home. I wanna go to bed!'

Chapter 15

While Jenson was upstairs in his room – sleeping or other-wise, I was happy to leave him up there to cool down for a bit – I called Riley to let her know about the change of plan.

'That's okay,' she said. 'I'll collect Levi from nursery and bring our picnic to yours. The boys won't care whether we're there or on the playing field. In fact, they'll probably prefer to be at yours – especially if you get the paddling pool out. No improvement on the Georgie–Jenson front, then?'

'Not on the Jenson front, to be sure,' I confirmed, and there must have been something extra-meaningful in my sigh, because Riley picked up on it immediately.

'Not like you to sound so negative, Mum,' she observed. 'God, I'd have thought that after Ashton and Olivia you could handle anything. Why's this kid getting to you so much?'

I sighed again. Ashton and Olivia seemed so long ago now, and in my current state – memory probably clouded – I didn't remember them being half so bad.

'I don't know. It's having the both of them together, I think, mainly. Georgie's complex, but actually he's no sort of bother, but having the two of them … I don't know. I just don't seem to be developing any sort of workable relationship with Jenson … We seem perpetually at loggerheads …'

'You mean that, basically, you don't like him.'

'God, no!'

'Mum, you know, you're not an angel or anything. It *is* within the bounds of possibility – albeit rarely – that you'll have a child in who you find hard to bond with. In fact, that's one of the things that got brought up at mine and David's last interview. They said it would be unrealistic to expect that you'd love *every* child that came into your care.' Riley paused to let this bit of wisdom sink in. 'Anyway,' she said finally, 'I'll let you go. I have a few errands to run before I come to you. Anything you need while I'm at the shops? Crate of valium? Case of gin?'

I laughed, of course, but Riley's words had cut me to the quick. She was right, yes, but me? Actively dislike a child I fostered? It had never happened. It couldn't happen. I refused to accept it. I'd dealt – both as a foster mum and as a school behaviour manager – with kids way more difficult to bond with than Jenson. No, it seemed more that he didn't bond with *me*. And thinking that made me feel pretty guilty as well, and reminded me that there must be a reason for Jenson's angry carapace. And I had yet to find it. With

Georgie joining us, I hadn't so far even *tried* that hard. And that made me feel bad as well.

But you can never feel bad for long when you have a brace of lovely grandchildren, and spending an hour in the company of mine worked its magic. By the time I had to go back to school to collect Georgie my sense of optimism had seeped back into my psyche as surely as the water from the paddling pool had seeped into my clothes.

And Georgie, too, seemed happy when he was returned to me. He'd spent the afternoon, with his teaching assistant, in a far-flung quiet classroom, building a small colourful citadel out of Lego. I'd recently learned that he really enjoyed both Lego and jigsaw puzzles, which was a bonus – something else to occupy him with while I dealt with Jenson.

But as he looked around now, he seemed slightly baffled. 'Good day,' he said, in response to my enquiry. 'But where is Jenson? Why is Jenson not here?'

'At home,' I explained. 'Nothing for you to worry about, sweetie. I'm afraid he's been naughty so Mrs Cappleman had to send him home.'

We were walking towards the car, but Georgie stopped dead on the pavement. 'Jenson naughty?' he said. Then shook his head. 'No. Jenson good. Jenson is good boy today.' He then looked down and began frowning, and I realised that as we'd approached the kerbside I had automatically held out my hand to him to cross.

I smiled bemusedly. How strange the rest of the world must seem to him. People trying to touch you and grab you and generally invade your space. I lowered my hand again, but then he surprised me. 'Not today,' he said. 'Maybe tomorrow I will hold it.' Then he glared. 'Jordan Gates is a motherfucker.'

'Georgie!' I gasped. 'That's a *bad* word to say. Where did you hear that? You mustn't say that word again, okay?'

'Jordan Gates is a motherfucker,' he said once again anyway. 'The opening episode of *Doctor Who* was called "An Unearthly Child". Susan had superior intelligence.'

Hmm, I thought. *And in some ways, so do you …*

Though, in some ways, he was as blank a mental slate as a baby. I wondered who'd thought it clever to teach him that word. Someone fairly close to home, I didn't doubt.

The number one candidate had come down when we returned home from school, and while Georgie went upstairs to change out of his uniform I watched the tableau in the garden through the kitchen window. It was actually fascinating to see how natural and happy Jenson was with the little ones, playing with them happily and attentively and carefully. Like a different child, in fact. He really was a puzzle. So much so that when he came inside to refill the jug of squash he even asked politely if Levi and Jackson could stay for tea.

'Of course they can,' I told him. 'If that suits Riley, that is. And as long as you all play nicely. Though, Jenson,' I added, as he went to get the squash bottle, 'no more teaching Georgie swear words, okay?'

I was pleased that the expected denial wasn't forthcoming on this occasion. In fact, he even had the grace to look sheepish. 'Oh, and Jenson,' I added, 'do you know who Jordan Gates is?'

He looked even more sheepish. 'He's a big bully. One of them boys I was fighting.' And after he'd fought them, also described them using his usual colourful language, no doubt. Which Georgie had obviously picked up on. But there was nothing to be gained by going over the same ground as earlier. Better to enjoy what remained of the afternoon with the little ones. Perhaps Jenson would open up to me about the incident in school this evening. Or perhaps not. Either way, it was best left right now. It would doubtless all come out in the wash.

In the event, it didn't. When I took Jenson to school the following morning I was none the wiser about the cause of the fight, because he flatly refused to discuss it, and I wondered if he was being bullied, perhaps about the situation at home. He had, after all, made reference to at least one of those involved being a bully himself. Perhaps his deputy head teacher would enlighten me.

But Andrea Cappleman, apparently, was also none the wiser, both the other boys having remained tight lipped about it, saying only that Jenson had wound them up.

'I'll keep an eye on things,' she told me. 'Though I don't doubt it'll blow over; these things usually do. Plus we *are* mindful that Jenson's in a bad place at the moment – which will of course make him extra wind-uppable.'

Though not, it seemed, so distressed that he didn't still find time to cause mischief of his own. That same afternoon, crossing the playground with Georgie, having picked him up, I was accosted by a lady I recognised. She was a dinner lady, and also the gran of one of the pupils, and was obviously here again to pick her up.

'Hello, Georgie,' she said, as we met in the middle of the playground. Then, looking at me pointedly, she continued. 'I'm glad to have bumped into you, because Georgie and I chatted at lunchtime, didn't we, Georgie? And Georgie asked me why I had whiskers on my chin.' If that didn't make we squirm – which it did: the poor woman – what she said next certainly did.

'And when I told him that was a rude thing to say,' the woman continued, 'Georgie's response was to say "Fuck off, whiskers!"'

Mortified and apologetic as I was to hear this, I did have a sneaking sympathy for Georgie, hearing this. After all, both he and the dinner lady had been at the school long enough for her to know Georgie was simply parroting something he'd heard, and I didn't doubt where he would have heard it either.

But when we got to the car, where Jenson was already waiting, my sympathy diminished somewhat when I realised Jenson had seen the exchange with the woman and that both boys were now giggling about it. I proffered the usual admonishments, of course. Ticked them both off for laughing and Georgie, in particular, for saying a rude word to the dinner lady. But even as I did so I realised that this was something of a breakthrough.

Because I had never heard Georgie laugh before, not once.

Georgie's unexpected giggles stayed with me for the rest of the day. Though it was clearly a bad thing that Jenson was using Georgie for his own entertainment in that way, I couldn't get over the shock of the emotional connection they had, for that moment, at least, seemed to make. It was a flimsy one, admittedly, and I still doubted Jenson's motivations, but when he asked me if they could go on a 'stone-hunting adventure' in the garden that Sunday morning I was prepared to give him the benefit of the doubt. Perhaps he was starting to accept Georgie after all.

'Of course you can,' I told him. 'What a brilliant idea. I might even come out and join in too, once I've peeled all this veg.'

'Can you believe that?' I said to Mike, as we watched them from out of the window. 'The two of them playing nicely together?'

'It was only a matter of time, love,' Mike said. 'They're kids, after all. It was probably as much about fighting for territory as anything. Although I wouldn't start counting your chickens just yet. They're just as likely to revert to fighting again.'

I smiled as I watched Jenson pick up a stone and polish it on his jeans before handing it to Georgie for inspection. Georgie did so, shook his head and Jenson took it back, shrugging, before tossing it back and looking for another. As simple pleasures went, it was pretty hard to knock.

And Mike was probably right. Jenson, forcibly removed from his home, had come to us and within a matter of a couple of weeks had been usurped by another child, and had to fight to keep his place in the pecking order. But maybe that had passed now – maybe they'd made enough of a connection that things between them would now begin to settle. And as for reverting, well, I could handle a little fall-out between them every now and again. That was to be expected with any kids.

The veg done, I rustled up some bacon and eggs for Mike. He'd had his one lie-in of the week, while I'd eaten breakfast with the boys, and it would be a good four or five hours before our roast. It was only once I'd done so and was washing my hands at the sink that I realised that, though Jenson was busy digging holes with a trowel still, there was no longer any sign of Georgie.

I called through the window. Perhaps he'd gone around the side path and I couldn't see him, or had come in to use the toilet while my back was turned.

'Where's Georgie, love?' I asked Jenson. He looked up and then around him. 'I dunno,' he said, shrugging. 'He was there a minute ago.' He got up off his knees and walked across to the side of the garden, where I joined him. It was then that I noticed that the gate, though shut, wasn't bolted. I felt a wave of panic wash over me. Georgie was not a child who had the skills to be out on the street alone. And he wouldn't be able to reach the bolt on his own, either. Probably wouldn't even think of trying, for that matter, unless …

'Did you unlock this?' I asked Jenson sharply.

'No!' he said. 'I *never*! I told you – I never saw him go out there!'

'He's not inside,' Mike said, joining us. 'I've been and checked upstairs.'

'So he's gone out into the street,' I said, pulling the gate open and dashing through it. It wasn't the busiest of locations where we lived now, plus it was Sunday, of course – but I couldn't help but think of the main road just a couple of streets away, and how easily Georgie might be panicked by the unfamiliarity of everything if he started wandering the streets alone.

Georgie, however, was nowhere to be seen. 'Right, young man,' I told Jenson, 'you stay right there in the garden, while Mike and I run to either end of the road.'

'I never done anything!' he bleated again. 'He just disappeared when I weren't looking!'

'I know, mate,' said Mike. 'You just hold the fort for thirty seconds. Casey, love,' he said, turning to me, 'I'll just head down to the junction, while you go that way. He'll not be far away, I'm sure.'

But our search on foot revealed no sign of him, and as we reconvened a minute later I felt a familiar sense of foreboding. We'd been here before – we'd had one child, Spencer, who could abscond for Great Britain, even via climbing out of a bedroom skylight and shimmying along roofs. But this was Georgie. Could he even cross a road unassisted? He was accompanied everywhere – into school, out of school, around school … And now we had absolutely no idea where he was.

'I'll go and get the car keys,' Mike said, squeezing my arm. 'And, love, stop panicking. We'll *find* him. It's only been minutes. He won't have got far.'

'What about the woods?' I said. 'Should Jenson and I go down to the woods, do you think?'

'Let me have a drive round first –' Mike stopped and glanced over my shoulder. 'Look, there's the Stanleys. Let's ask if they might have seen him.'

The Stanleys were our next-door neighbours and were coming down the road, presumably returning home from church. But they'd seen no sign of Georgie, and as they went into their house and Mike jumped in the car to go and look for him I felt surer than ever that he might have wandered down to the woods. We'd talked about them, after all, and how he might well find some stones there.

'Think,' I said to Jenson, wondering if he'd suggested that very thing. 'What might you have said that would make him go off like that?'

'*Nothing!*' he said. 'Honest, Casey. I didn't say nothing to him. Not a word!'

I was just scrabbling for my door keys, having decided to head across the park anyway, when an ear-splitting scream rent the still Sunday air. A Georgie-scream, and clearly close at hand. Relief coursed through me. But where was he then? Somewhere to the left. I went back down the side path to the front, where, looking down the alleyway that separated our two houses, I saw Mr Stanley tugging a panicked Georgie along by his hand.

'Oh, let him go!' I cried, much to Mr Stanley's confusion. 'That's why he's screaming. You mustn't touch him. He doesn't like it …'

Mr Stanley seemed only too happy to oblige. Georgie stopped dead then, shook his fringe from his eyes, and did his cupped-hands thing; staring down at what looked like an ordinary bunch of pebbles, but clearly one that meant a great deal to him, because as Mr Stanley leaned down to see what Georgie was holding he clasped his hands together around them and promptly began screaming again.

'Georgie, come on,' I said, thinking on my feet now. His collection tin was sitting on our patio table, wasn't it? 'Come on. That's obviously a *very* important stone for your collection so you need to go back into our garden and put it safely in your tin.'

This seemed to do the trick. Clutching his hands straight out in front of him, he marched straight past me and Jenson, and inside the garden gate with his all-important new treasure.

'I didn't hurt him, my love,' Mr Stanley said, looking bewildered. 'I'm sure I didn't. I was just worried he might make a dash for it, that's all.'

It was only the work of moments to put our poor next-door neighbour in the picture. And it seemed that Georgie had been in their garden all along. They'd come home and gone inside and nearly jumped out of their skins to see a small boy in their garden, kneeling down in front of their ornamental rockery, having excavated a sizeable hole.

'Which is no bother at all,' Mr Stanley assured me, when I explained about Georgie's collection of 'precious' stones and what they meant to him. 'So don't you worry. I'm just glad to know the lad is safely found.'

And he wasn't the only one. It was a good quarter of an hour before Mike returned. Stupidly, neither of us had thought that it might be an idea for him to take a mobile.

'But no harm done,' we agreed, as he joined us in the garden, where Georgie was reconfiguring a new row of stones. Seeing Mike, he glanced up, and then picked one of the new stones up. Then he pointed to Jenson. 'Rock-er-y. Grey-green. For you,' he said.

Both Mike and my eyes moved to Jenson.

'Grey-green for Jenson,' Georgie said again. 'Cream-white for Georgie. Georgie is a clever boy,' he finished.

Jenson's mouth fell open. 'I never!' he said. 'I never said for him to go there!'

'So why did he?' I asked him.

'I never said to! I didn't!'

At which point Georgie started up all over again. 'Jenson said! Jenson said! Georgie clever!' he kept repeating, between screams.

I turned to Jenson, conscious of the appalling racket we were creating. 'Just go upstairs,' I told him, 'while we try to calm him down, will you?'

And as Jenson ran past me, his look of outrage was so powerful that it was a miracle I didn't fall down on the spot.

* * *

Predictably, once Jenson had gone, Georgie did stop. And once again it happened as abruptly as it started. He put the stones down on the table, again – one at the end of the row he'd just created, and one slightly aside – the one for Jenson. That done, he then began picking them up again, one by one, and placing them, in some seemingly random but probably exact order, in his tin.

'Sweetheart, you mustn't go out of the garden on your own,' I told him. 'Do you understand? It's dangerous for Georgie to go out alone.'

'Dangerous,' Georgie said, nodding, though still absorbed in making adjustments. 'Rockery dangerous. Georgie understands.'

'Anyway,' said Mike, 'all's well that ends well. You get your collection back upstairs, lad, and perhaps we'll all of us go on a nice walk to the woods, eh?'

I watched as Georgie trotted back inside, oblivious to the emotional chaos he had created. Or, rather, that had been created *around* him.

'Nice walk in the woods?' I said. 'Nice? You know, I *knew* it. I knew it was too good to be true. He's obviously sent him over to next door's garden on purpose, so –'

'He?'

'Jenson,' I said. 'He's obviously put him up to it, hasn't he?'

I stopped speaking, because Mike was looking at me strangely. 'Love, can you hear yourself?' he said. 'Hear what you're saying? Jenson is 9. How can he possibly understand the danger of Georgie going outside on his own?'

I took this in, and was shocked. 'Hang on. Are you saying you *don't* think Jenson put him up to this?'

'No, I'm not saying he did or he didn't. We don't know. Just that he wouldn't have known the implications – *or* the danger. And it seems to me that you're being just a little too quick to blame him.'

'No, I'm not,' I said, gobsmacked. 'I'm just not being naïve. And, if you ask me, this only goes to reinforce what I've been thinking. That it's not going to be possible for me to care for Georgie properly while we still have Jenson living with us as well.'

Mike's expression changed to one that I'd seen many times before. 'Love,' he said, 'don't take this the wrong way or anything, but don't you think you might be overcompensating just a little?'

'Overcompensating?'

'Yes, for Kieron.'

'What on earth does Kieron have to do with it?'

'I'm just saying that perhaps you're being a bit overprotective with Georgie, because you worry that you didn't always get it right when Kieron was his age and –'

'Mike, that's patent nonsense! I'm just being realistic. Georgie has special needs, and I'm struggling to get my head around them –'

And then came the look again, which was a bit like a slap around the face with a wet flannel. 'And what, love? Jenson's getting in the way?'

Chapter 16

After what Mike had said to me I spent the whole night tossing and turning. Was I being too hard on Jenson? My head said I wasn't. He'd obviously come from a place without discipline and, though he was in a difficult situation – which would obviously affect his behaviour – I was clear that we would be doing him no favours whatsoever if we failed to provide strict boundaries for him. That was our job as foster carers, surely?

But Mike's comment, that I favoured Georgie and was perhaps seeing Jenson as 'being in the way', rankled. I was only human, and I obviously had a soft spot for poor Georgie, so of course I got upset when Jenson tormented him. But perhaps *too* upset? I decided to hold off asking John about moving him; I would hate that anyone thought I was showing favouritism between the boys.

It was clear that Jenson thought exactly that, as well. When I dropped the boys at school the following morning he didn't say goodbye to me; but then, he didn't really need to – the way he slammed the car door and marched off up the school drive told me everything I needed to know. And even worse was that Georgie seemed to want to shun me now as well. He had to walk with me, of course – I always took him right in to school, to his teaching assistant – but he seemed determined to stride off in front, as if disowning me, much more anxious to catch up with Jenson.

Being a foster parent – being any parent – isn't about being popular, but being this *un*popular still brought me down. And when I returned home I knew I'd probably bring myself down even further – I decided I would call John in any case. Quite apart from anything else, we were still in the dark about when – or if – this emergency 'few days' placement (now several weeks in) was likely to come to an end. Which was not at all – I told myself – about us wanting to see Jenson gone, but all about him wanting to go home.

But there was nothing positive to report. 'I'm really sorry, Casey,' John said, 'but it's still a work in progress, I'm afraid. How's it going anyway? Must be challenging, looking after a boy like Georgie, even for an expert like you. Are you and Mike managing to cope with him okay?'

I actually had to bite my lip, hearing that, for fear of adopting a holier-than-thou tone with him. I really liked and respected John, and, to be fair, why would he think any differently about Georgie? He was autistic, which *was* challenging, but while my head was busy thinking that, my heart had swelled over with a great wash of angry defensiveness, which had come out of nowhere. Couldn't he see it? It was Jenson who was the one causing the problems!

I gave myself a moment before answering more rationally. 'Oh, not too bad,' I said lightly, 'considering the mix we have. We've had our moments with the pair of them, as you can imagine.'

'I *can* imagine,' said John. 'And you've been a brick to have both of them. And I know Marie is doing her utmost to sort things out. Set up another contact visit, at the very least. And it's so annoying – were it not for this fiancé moving in, we would have had the kids both home with Mum two weeks ago.'

Which was all too depressingly familiar a scenario. 'Do we know any more about him?'

'I don't personally,' said John, 'but it seems things have come up on his police check. Things involving violence. Which of course creates an issue.' He sighed. 'It's the same old balancing act, Casey, as per always; weighing up the likely risk of him offending again ...'

'And what if they decide the risk's too high?'

'Then it's Karen's choice, obviously. Let's just hope it doesn't come to that, eh?'

So it was a 'cross that bridge when we come to it' scenario. It often was. And if it did come to that, it would be Karen who made that choice. Choose the fiancé over getting her kids home? For almost everyone that would be a no-brainer. But, sadly, I'd been around long enough to know the way the world worked. There *were* women who would choose the fiancé.

I put the phone down on John with my mood just as low. Which meant there was only one thing for it. Do some cleaning. Some might consider it the raving lunacy of a mad woman, but I knew the best antidote to an uncharacteristically gloomy mindset was, for me, at least, the donning of Marigolds, the application of some elbow grease, and the smell of cleaning fluids pricking at my nostrils.

By Monday afternoon my house was so spotless it positively thrummed; so much so that by Wednesday, when Kieron came round for tea, brimming with 'big big' news (as we liked to say in our house), he could still smell the whiff of solvents in the air.

'You know, Mum,' he observed, 'when people talk about the smell that most reminds them of home, almost all of them will say the smell of coffee brewing, or a cake baking, or a roast dinner in the oven, but for me it will always be Mr Muscle.' He clasped a hand to his chest theatrically. 'Ah, home,' he trilled 'where the evocative scent of toilet bleach mingles so beautifully with the sweet scent of window and glass cleaner, offset by a pleasing top note of super-action bathroom mousse.'

I gave him a playful slap. 'Okay, so that's your big big news then, is it? That you've got yourself a place at RADA? Stop taking the mick, you meanie! Come on, spill the beans. What's the news, really?'

Big, as it turned out. Very big, in fact. Kieron – to my great pride – had managed to bag himself a voluntary position as a trainee teaching assistant at a local primary school, no less. And one in which they would also pay his college fees, so that he could work towards a formal qualification as a teaching assistant as well.

'And they even said there would be a position for me there at the end of it,' he enthused. 'A proper paid one. Isn't that great?'

'Absolutely brilliant,' I agreed. But at the same time I wasn't naïve. I knew it would be a lot for him to take on. I was so proud of my son, and how he'd overcome his challenges, but I was also concerned that he didn't get so carried away that he took on too much at once and overdid it. He already had his youth-centre football team to manage, plus his part-time job at my sister's café, to help make ends meet. Which was a lot to be juggling, even if you were a strapping young man. Particularly one who was so easily stressed.

But Kieron was predictably optimistic about how he'd cope. 'Stop worrying, Mum,' he chided. 'I have it all worked out. I've already spoken to Auntie Donna, and she said she'll re-jig my shifts around my school days, and football's in the evenings, so there's no problem there.'

I was just about to remind him about not stretching himself so far that he'd get fed up – with my years in the comprehensive behind me, I knew just how much a 'short' school day could take it out of you – when we were interrupted by a commotion coming from the living room.

We both looked through to see Georgie rocking wildly on the sofa, intermittently screaming and shouting 'No,

Jenson, no, Jenson!' while flapping his arms nine to the dozen.

'Honestly!' I said to Kieron, marching to open the French doors that separated us and the boys. 'I can't leave them alone for five minutes before Jenson starts winding Georgie up!'

Which he was clearly doing right now. As I entered the room I could now see him, and see that he was pulling faces, to boot.

'Jenson,' I snapped. 'Knock it off, will you!'

'But it's him!' Jenson answered, the usual defiant look on his face. 'He's being a weirdo again, staring at me and laughing at me for no reason!'

'Oh, for goodness sake,' I said. '*How* old are you? Old enough to be able to ignore something so silly. And anyway,' I went on, placing a hand on each hip, 'why is *he* the one shouting "no", then? And how many times must I tell you not to call him that, Jenson? For goodness' sake. Do you *want* him to kick off? Is that it?'

'But he *is* a weirdo!' he persisted. 'An' he creeps me out! An' he's saying "no" because I keep telling him to stop it and leave me alone!'

I looked across at Georgie, who, quiet now, seemed to be taking this all in. And, yes, he was indeed staring at Jenson. But as soon as he realised I was looking at him, he started whooping and flapping and saying 'No, Jenson!' again.

'Shh, Georgie,' I said. 'Come on, now. Enough of this noise. And you,' I said, turning back to Jenson irritably, 'for goodness' sake just *ignore* him. I have to get tea now and I'd be grateful for a little bit less noise.'

I turned to go back into the kitchen. 'What about *him*?' Jenson spluttered. 'Why aren't you telling *him* off? Why aren't you telling *him* to stop staring at me and being all weird?!'

'I just *did*,' I said. 'I –'

'No you didn't. You didn't *blame* him. You blamed *me*!'

'Jenson –' I began. Then I thought better of it. Being blamed was a big thing with Jenson – especially after Sunday. So it would serve no useful purpose to fan that particular fire again now. 'And you too, Georgie,' I said, turning to him and gently waggling a finger. 'No more staring at Jenson, okay, mister?'

Georgie blinked at me. I had absolutely no idea if anything had registered. But that wasn't the point. The important thing was that Jenson had heard it, so he could balance that tally of rebukes in his head.

'Right,' I said to Kieron, closing the French doors again. 'Where were we?'

'Honestly, Mum,' he chuckled. 'You do get worked up over the silliest things.'

'*What*?' I blustered. 'You should try living in this mad house, believe me! Anyway. It's not silly. There's nothing big or clever about calling someone a weirdo, Kieron. You, of all people, should understand that. It's not nice and I'm sick of hearing it, frankly.'

'Honest, Mum. You're too sensitive. Kids used to call me that all the time at school.'

'Don't I know it!'

'Yeah, but that's just the *point*, Mum. You'd get all upset about it, but I didn't care. I *was* weird, compared to them. And they seemed pretty weird to me, as well.'

'Kieron, you are not "weird".'

'But I *am*, Mum. Of course I am.' He looked at me as if I had lost all my marbles. 'Don't you remember what that doctor said? That one up at the hospital? All that stuff about me being special, because my brain was wired up differently to other kids' brains? And how it was because of that that I had all my funny little ways?' Kieron grinned. 'He was cool, that doctor. I really liked him for saying that.'

I was stunned at Kieron's recall. That was exactly what the doctor *had* said. And while I had sat there, listening to all the gentle euphemisms, and seeing only challenges and trials and potential problems for my lovely little boy, Kieron had seen things completely differently. Kieron had felt special and understood.

'You shouldn't get so het up about it, Mum,' he finished. 'I know kids shouldn't call other kids names, but to Jenson Georgie *is* weird. Scary-weird – much more scary-weird than I was. And trust me, when he does that look of his he even scares me! But he doesn't care. I bet you. He doesn't care at all. *I* never did. You did. But I didn't.'

And, God, I did remember. Could remember it as if it were yesterday. How aware I was of other mums whisper-ing about him, how much it hurt when there was yet another party he wasn't invited to, how much I felt the stares or the giggles or just the plain rejection of it all. My son, the odd one. The outcast. The one no one wanted to play with. Yet Kieron was right. I cared. But he didn't. He didn't want to play with any of the other kids anyway. Because they wouldn't play the games he wanted, wouldn't play the *way* he wanted; he'd always rather play alone, with all his 'funny little ways'.

And he'd been happy. And nothing had changed, really. He'd come such a long way, growing up, had such a fine set of social skills now. And as long as no one messed with his possessions or his routines, Kieron was as happy as the day was long.

And he was also right. Having Jenson and Georgie together was like picking at a scab that had long since healed over – so much that I forgot that I still bore the scar. I was looking at Georgie, and I was always seeing Kieron.

And my son wasn't finished with his homily. 'You're probably making it worse, Mum, to be honest. I'll bet Georgie doesn't care. But I bet Jenson does. He probably thinks you like Georgie more than him. And that makes him worse.'

I reached for the kettle. I needed caffeine. Not to mention a rap across the knuckles. 'You know what, babes?' I said to my annoyingly sagacious son. 'You're right. It pains me to admit it. But you're spot on.'

It seemed incredible to me that ten minutes with Kieron could alter my perspective so dramatically, though having had it altered I felt a great deal better about myself. A great deal better, come to that, about our little mismatched family, and in particular about poor, beleaguered Jenson.

Kieron had hit the nail on the head – Georgie wasn't 'hurt' by being teased. Georgie was only hurt by having his physical space invaded, by people trying to make eye contact with him, and by people interfering with or changing his routine. The word 'weirdo' sloughed off him like rain off a windscreen. It simply didn't register. He didn't have the emotional intelligence. He was, in fact, the living embodiment of the phrase *sticks and stones may break my bones but names will never hurt me*.

And, if to a slightly lesser extent (I didn't doubt Kieron could have his heart broken, for instance) Kieron, with his mild Asperger's, was the same. He could only see the good in people; with only a slight grasp on emotional complexity, he had no reason to see anything in other than concrete terms. If someone called him 'weird', it was just a word – a statement of fact to him. A statement, moreover, that he agreed with – unencumbered by any notions of someone 'being unkind'. He was wired one way, they were wired another. They were in the majority, so he was weird.

And Georgie, being a great deal further along the spectrum than Kieron, didn't even *use* vocabulary in the way 'normal' people did. In that, and every sense, his requirements to be 'happy' were simple: to feel safe, to have his needs met, to have no one invade that precious space. He had never known family life, so there was no way he could miss it – whereas Jenson, however erratic his parenting, had very much known it, and missed it, and felt bereft.

All of which I knew. But had forgotten. Temporarily.

Friday was Mike's birthday, and, feeling much happier about the boys now, I decided I would organise a babysitter for them and plan a much-needed family night out. Since our own kids would be coming with us, and I didn't want to call in a stranger, I asked my sister if she'd step in for a few hours. Like Kieron and Riley, she'd been police checked for just this kind of situation, and I knew that if anyone could handle my pair of chalk and cheese 9-year-olds, my no-nonsense capable sis definitely could.

So I was surprised to see her expression as we walked up the front path. We'd had a fabulous couple of hours, stuffing our faces with tortillas and enchiladas and, in the birthday boy's case, a steak the size of a breadboard. But the jolly air was obviously about to be overturned. She was looking out of the living room window, clearly relieved to see us back. Not like my sister at all.

'I didn't call,' she whispered, letting us in before Mike could even pull his key out, 'because I didn't want to spoil your evening. But, well –' she nodded, gesturing behind her, towards the living room. 'We've had a right carry-on with this one tonight.'

We glanced in, to where Jenson was curled up on the sofa, asleep but fully dressed, and puffy eyed.

'Been in a right state,' Donna explained, once we were out of earshot in the kitchen, and having established that

Georgie was fast asleep in bed. 'Started not long after you left. I could hear some noise upstairs – nothing worrying, or anything; I just assumed they were playing – but I obviously went up to check on them. Anyway, Georgie was in Jenson's bedroom, lining up those pebbles you mentioned – you know, the ones from his tin – sitting in the doorway, not doing anything much of anything, really, but Jenson clearly didn't want him there and started kicking off.'

'Oh, sis, I'm so sorry –' I began. But Donna shook her head.

'No, not like that. Not *at* Georgie or anything. He was just upset. Just in a proper state about where you'd gone and when you'd be home. And he's not really stopped since. Well, not till he flaked out – couldn't keep his eyes open. He was just in a right state about when you'd be home.'

Mike and I exchanged looks. Now this *was* weird. If there was one 9-year-old you wouldn't expect to worry about being home alone, it was Jenson. I said as much to Donna. It just didn't add up.

'What about Georgie?' asked Mike. 'Did he start kicking off as well?'

Donna shook her head. 'Not at all. Seemed in his own little world, he did. Once I went in to try and calm Jenson down, he just took himself and his stones off to bed. It was Jenson that was the problem; when I told him for the umpteenth time that I wasn't going to call you and cut short your evening, he got himself all dressed, coat on and everything, and when I tried to lock the door he even tried to make a run for it with the house phone so he could call your mobile – though where he thought he'd get the number from, I don't know!'

'Oh, you poor thing,' I said. 'Sounds like you've had a bit of a nightmare of an evening.'

Donna shook her head. 'I've had worse. Besides, had to do it for my lovely bro-in-law, didn't I? And we got there in the end – I brought him round with chocolate biscuits. He's been through a packet and a half, I'm afraid.'

'Oh, I don't think we'll worry about that,' I said. Recalling our recent trip to A&E, I was just relieved it hadn't been any worse.

'Hey, but on a more serious note, I did allow him half an hour on the laptop. Did you know about his obsession for NHS Direct?'

'*What*?' Mike said.

'He does seem to have something of a thing for weird websites. That one, as I say. And one about heart massage, of all things. St John's Ambulance. Certainly different. Perhaps he wants to be a paramedic when he grows up!'

After Donna had gone, Mike carried a still dozy Jenson upstairs, while I followed behind, carrying my strappy sandals. Between us we got Jenson into his pyjamas and into bed. Donna had been right. He'd done something of a 'rock star in a five-star hotel room' job on his bedroom. Though with no television to throw out of the window, it had escaped major damage; nothing that couldn't be sorted in the morning.

We left Jenson's door ajar and went to get into our own night things – it was quite late now – but just as I crossed the landing to go down and make a hot drink for the pair of us I heard him whisper to me from his room, in a small voice.

'Hey, sweetie,' I said, pushing the door open and looking in. 'We're home now. Go to sleep. We can talk in the morning.'

'You're not going out again?'

At midnight? *As if*, I thought. But then who knew what kinds of times Jenson's mother came and went? 'No,' I said. 'We're going to sleep. Which is what you should be doing.'

'I can't,' he said plaintively. 'My brain won't go to sleep now.'

I went in and sat on the bed. Jenson immediately sat up. 'Hey,' I said, putting my arms out. He immediately threw his own around me, surprising me. Since Georgie's arrival he'd backed off in that regard. I hugged him, feeling guilty. 'What is it, love?' I asked him softly. 'What was this evening all about then?'

'You left me,' he said immediately, clutching me tighter. 'You went out and left me.'

'Only for a meal, love,' I said. 'And Donna was here, wasn't she?'

'But you don't normally leave me,' he persisted.

'I know,' I said. 'Because we don't get out much. And don't *want* to,' I added. 'Just now and again, for special occasions.' I hugged him tighter, remembering his web search for first-aid scenarios. It felt peculiar, but perhaps he really *was* fearful of being left. 'But if I'd known you were going to be so scared, love …' I started.

'I wasn't scared!' came the immediate retort, with a fair degree of feeling. 'But you shouldn'a left me in charge of Georgie. It's not fair! What if the social found out? What if the social come and saw it?'

I pulled back a little to look at him. 'Why on earth would they do that, love? You had a babysitter. She was here to look after you *and* Georgie –'

'An' then they'd take me away again,' he said, obviously not listening to my answer. 'An' I'd have to go an' live somewhere else again, cos they'd say it was my fault!'

'But love …'

'You shouldn'a left me to take care of him.'

'But we didn't, Jenson. We'd never do that. That wouldn't be responsible. That wouldn't be *fair*.'

'Don' matter,' he said. 'If owt had happened I'd get the blame for it.'

'Of course you wouldn't, love. It's –'

'Yeah, I *would*,' he said doggedly. 'Just like I did about our Sammy.'

I looked at him. I was obviously onto something here. Sammy? 'Jenson,' I said. 'Who's Sammy?'

He looked back at me, and I saw panic cross his features. So I said it again. 'Jenson, who's Sammy?'

It was dark in Jenson's room, but there was light enough to see the fear. 'No one,' he said, pulling away. 'No one!'

Chapter 17

If someone says someone is 'no one', particularly if that someone is a child, then it's odds on that the someone is someone quite important – and in this case I'd have bet my last farthing on the fact.

I woke up, bleary-eyed, to see the clock display in front of me. It read 09:51. Almost ten! But it wasn't surprising. When you spend half the night wide awake, engaged in thinking about such tongue-twisting conundrums, it's no wonder you oversleep the next morning.

I rolled over. Mike's side of the bed was empty, as expected. It being a Saturday, he'd have already been down to the warehouse for an hour, and if my nostrils didn't deceive me – I sniffed, no they didn't – well under way with preparing breakfast.

Time to get up, then. I swung my legs out of bed and pushed my feet into my slippers. It already looked like being a beautiful sunny day. And who knew? Perhaps one without any crises or dramas. Miracles did sometimes happen, after all.

And when I got downstairs, things certainly looked hopeful in that department. The dining-room table had already been laid, complete with morning paper and my favourite brown sauce, while Mike himself, assisted by both Jenson and Georgie, was busy dishing up plates of bacon and scrambled eggs. I noticed Jenson looked a little puffy-eyed. Perhaps he'd had a wakeful night as well. He glanced across at me and gave me a wan smile.

'That's what I like to see,' I said, smiling back as I took my place at the table. 'Men at work! God, that smells delicious.'

'Georgie is going to football today,' Georgie told me, taking his place beside me and carefully putting down his plate of scrambled eggs with barely toasted toast.

I glanced across at Mike as Jenson came to the table with his own breakfast. This was a first.

Mike nodded. 'We're all going to go and watch Kieron, aren't we, kiddo? That's if you didn't have any other plans for these two,' he said to me. 'He's only playing just up the road, so I thought we could all stroll up there together. Lovely day for it, after all. Anyway, tuck in.'

I loved that Mike was being so proactive with them both, though I did have plans, as it happened. Well, one plan, at any rate. To find a way to get Jenson to open up about who this 'Sammy' was. It didn't take a degree in rocket science to come up with the possibility that the name Sammy and the neighbour's comment about 'all that business with the little one' might be connected in some way. But in what way, exactly? That was the question.

'That sounds like a lovely idea,' I agreed, squeezing a big dollop of sauce on to my plate. 'And best of all, it'll give me a chance to top up my tan. Except ...' I added, thinking on my slippered feet, like a pro. 'Before you do that, I have to nip into town and pick up a couple of bits and bobs for Riley, and I was hoping you might come with me, Jenson.' I turned to face him. 'I promised Levi we'd get some of that new pirate-ship Lego, and I thought you might like to help me choose it. And there was that DS game you fancied, wasn't there? The one about ...'

'The penguins!' Jenson said, his eyes lighting up on cue. 'Could I get that?'

I nodded, pleased at the simplicity of a young boy's mental wiring. 'I don't see why not. And something for Georgie, as well. Since you both helped make us such a lovely breakfast. And once we're done, I could drop you off at the playing fields to join Mike and Georgie to watch the match, couldn't I?' I turned to Mike. 'Would that be a plan, love?' I asked him.

He winked. He had clearly worked out mine.

In my experience, car journeys always seem to be good environments in which to have discussions. Particularly discussions about difficult subjects. And particularly discussions involving children. I don't know why it is, but it always seems to be so. Perhaps it's the calming environment. Perhaps it's because you don't need to make eye contact. Or perhaps it's just because neither party has the opportunity to walk away if things get too sensitive or too heated. It always worked with my own kids – and particularly when they were stroppy teenagers. Yes, we'd always end with them slamming the door and stomping off in a huff, but not before absorbing whatever homily about homework or housework or acceptable coming-home times was on the mum-agenda that day.

Jenson wasn't a teenager, stroppy or otherwise, but based on his reaction to my probing the night before I didn't imagine he would open up that readily about what the significance of this 'Sammy' person was. I also had a hunch – again, not rocket science, really – that it was something that troubled him deeply. What had happened? What kind of 'bad business' had gone on? Had he hurt another kid? Or been involved in some kind of childish crime? Was this 'Sammy' an accomplice? It could be so many things. But one thing was a definite. It was a burden.

I decided I would broach it on the way back from shopping, rather than on the way there. Thrilled with his new game (which he was; he was sitting in the back seat, reading the back of it) he might feel more disposed to open up to me. Low tactics – I was in full-on Lieutenant Columbo mode by this time – but, hopefully, a valid means to an end. I really wanted to know what ailed this complicated child, because something did. And my hunch was that it was more than just erratic parenting.

'Jenson,' I asked him lightly, as we left the multi-storey car park. 'You know when we were talking last night?'

He glanced up from his reading, looking wary.

'Well, you know, sweetheart, it's been on my mind ever since. I can't help wondering. What happened? Who *is* Sammy?'

I could see his face in the rear-view mirror, and how it changed. 'No one. I *told* you,' he said, staring fixedly at the game box.

'Sweetheart, everyone is *someone*,' I said. 'No one can be no one. Is he a friend of yours? Someone you know? Someone you knew?'

'I told you,' he said again. '*No one!*'

He stared at my reflection in the mirror now, as if to will me to leave it by the power of a glare alone. Which made me all the more determined that leaving it was what I shouldn't do. 'Why won't you tell me, love?' I asked him mildly. 'Is it something you find difficult to –'

'I *can't!*' he said, looking exasperated now. 'I mustn't!'

'But why?' I asked. 'Sweetheart, whatever it is, I'm sure you'll feel better if you get it off your chest.'

'But it's a secret!' His tone was now becoming pleading. '*Please*, Casey. I should never of said it. I should never of said her name!'

Despite my desire to get to the bottom of this, I knew I had to be careful. Much as I knew that getting to the truth was one of the best ways you could help heal a troubled child, I was also part of a social-service system which had clearly defined protocols and boundaries. Which was a good thing – following procedure protected us from both criticism and lawsuits – but it could also be frustrating, particularly when it stopped me from doing what I always wanted to; having a full and open relationship with the children in my care. And it had only recently got me into trouble as well. Our last foster child's mother had harboured a big secret, and when I found out about it and confronted her, it didn't matter a jot that it changed everything for the better – I still got my knuckles rapped for not following protocol. Even though I felt I'd done the right thing – and still did – by the book I still shouldn't have done it. I should have taken my concerns to her social worker and left her to deal with it, rather than trying to sort it out myself.

So this was delicate ground. Where there were secrets, there were generally lies. Whatever this secret was, it wasn't likely to be a nice one.

'A secret?' I asked lightly, noting that Sammy was female. 'Whose secret, sweetheart?'

This seemed to faze him.

'I mean, who told you to keep it secret, love? Was it Sammy? Because if she's done something to upset you and asked you to keep it a secret, then that's not right, love, is it?'

We'd stopped at traffic lights by now, so I twisted round to look at him directly. And in doing so, I noticed that his eyes had filled with tears. This was beginning to feel too much like an interrogation. Which was the last thing I wanted. If he felt he really couldn't talk, then it would be wrong to push it. But that was the most frustrating thing. If it really was that upsetting, then it *was* a big thing. A huge thing he was carrying around all by himself.

But just as I'd decided to leave it – perhaps I *would* just speak to Marie about it, after all – Jenson spoke again. 'It weren't Sammy,' he answered, crying now. 'How could it be Sammy? She were only little.' He took a gulp of air. 'She din't do nothing! An' she's dead! An' you shouldn'a asked me, Casey. Mum'll go apeshit! An' it'll all be *your* fault!'

Finding a place to pull over took a good five minutes. And all the while, Jenson sat and wept in the back seat, arms crossed across his chest, the penguin DS game clamped between them, his face wrestling with itself as he tried to stem the flow.

Finally I managed to park, and swivelled right round in the front seat. Then, deciding that this wouldn't do, I climbed out of the car and got back into the back seat, beside him.

'Sweetheart,' I said softly, as he sat rigidly beside me. 'I hate seeing you so upset. It's just that –'

'I'm not upset!' came the immediate retort. 'I'm just cross! You'd shouldn' keep on at me. Getting me in trouble. I'm not allowed to tell!'

'Tell what?'

'About my sister!'

'Carley?'

'No, *Sammy*!'

'Sammy's your sister?' I backtracked. No. Wrong. *Was* his sister. 'Sammy was your sister? Your little sister? And she died?'

Jenson nodded miserably. 'Casey, *please* don't tell on me. My mum will go mad. She will. She'll go *apeshit* if she knows I said owt to anyone. Promise you won't? Cross your heart?'

My brain was now in overdrive. No wonder this was a big thing for him – whatever this 'thing' actually was. But I reined myself in. There was nothing to be gained right now by trying to dig up any more. Right now he clearly needed reassurance that he wasn't in trouble.

'Sweetheart, of *course* I won't say anything to your mum. I wouldn't dream of it. And of course you're not in trouble. Why on earth would you be in trouble? I won't say a word to her, I promise. Not a word.'

'Promise?'

'Cross my heart,' I said, making the gesture twice, for good measure.

It didn't take long then for Jenson to stop crying and wipe his face. And it struck me how this wasn't so much about the pain of loss, but about fear. He was mostly just terrified of me telling on him and getting him into trouble with his mother. Which naturally begged the question – *why*?

I tried to unscramble my memories of what he'd said the previous evening. Blame. He'd said something about being always blamed for everything. And unjustly. It had always been something of a theme with him. But, once again, why? What was the big secret around his little sister's death? Why had he been ordered by his mum to keep it quiet?

While Jenson returned to looking at his game, my mind was full of questions. Questions like a bunch of Lego bricks, all in a muddle, and which needed piecing together to make a coherent whole. But what would it look like? Odds on, pretty ugly.

With coffee, half an hour later, came clarity. By the time we'd arrived at the football field Jenson had seemed much happier. Happy just to get out of my car, was my guess. Happy to run to Mike and Georgie. Happy to watch Kieron play football. Happy not to be interrogated by me any further, mainly. Which was something of a relief, because the last thing I wanted was to cause him any further distress.

But I still wanted answers, because it was all such a mystery. Precisely what was Jenson's mother so keen to keep buried? And more chilling than that, should this be a police matter? I was all too aware that her fiancé was currently being police-checked. Was this something to do with him? And just when had all this happened? Was I now privy to information about a murder?

I probably would have got into a bit of a flap at this point were it not for the fact that logic quickly prevailed. Whatever 'it' was, it was out there. It almost certainly was out there. What the neighbour – Mrs Clark – had said corroborated that. She'd talked about a bad business with a little one, hadn't she? Something like that, anyway, I thought, gulping down my coffee. And then it hit me. I had her number. So why didn't I just call her?

Getting my phone out of my handbag, I did a mental run-through of the protocol. Would I be breaking any if I spoke to her? I didn't see how. We'd swapped numbers, after all, and it wasn't as if I was doing anything underhand. She'd started to tell me something that day and all I was doing now was hearing the rest of it.

No, I thought, pressing the 'call contact' key. It would be fine.

And happily, she was in and prepared to talk to me. Very keen to talk to me, in fact: I got the distinct impression that not only did she love a gossip, but also that this was a subject about which she felt quite strongly.

'Oh, the poor mite,' she said, once I'd explained I was calling about Jenson, and how he'd alluded to his little sister's death. 'Poor mite,' she said again. 'Such a terrible business. I'm surprised you didn't know about it. Didn't the girl from the social tell you? It's not as if it isn't common knowledge, after all. Was in all the papers. On the telly news as well.'

So that was one worry dealt with. I wasn't party to some sort of hideous cover-up. But what Mrs Clark had to tell me was pretty hideous even so.

'Drowned, she did, little Sammy. Aged 2 at the time. And only just, as well. I remember that in particular because one of the things that stuck in my mind, reading the paper, was how she'd got the paddling pool for her second birthday.'

'She drowned?'

'That's what the coroner said. Accidental death due to drowning. She somehow fell into the paddling pool while Jenson was indoors looking for lollies. I don't know all the exact details, but that was the gist of it.' She sighed. 'Just like they always tell you, isn't it? That a little one can drown in just a couple of inches of water. I think she might have slipped and banged her head … as I say, I don't know all the details. But that's how she found her when she came back from the shop.'

I was thrown. 'When who came back? Jenson's mother? Karen?'

'Yes, dear. That's the whole point. She wasn't there. She'd left them. That's the scandal of it – that she left him – poor Jenson. No more than 5, he was. And she left him minding her. Carley was off playing round a friend's house, so she just left them. Left a 5-year-old in charge of a tot like that while she was off buying her ciggies at the corner shop. Couldn't be bothered to get the buggy out, most probably, knowing her. Can you credit it? I can't. Never could. Oh, you should have heard the screams that day, believe me. Went right through me.'

'Oh my God,' I said, trying to imagine. Which I couldn't. And I sincerely hoped I never would have to. What a terrible, senseless loss. What a tragedy. And what an awful thing for Jenson to have to live with. What a weight for a child to have to bear.

I told Mrs Clark about how frightened Jenson was that I might tell his mother what he'd told me. How it was a secret that Karen had told him he mustn't tell. How he wasn't even supposed to mention his little sister's name. Mrs Clark snorted at this. Actually snorted.

'*Secret*? How does she make that one stick? Don't make

me laugh. But it doesn't surprise me. Course she doesn't want him blabbing. Telling strangers. Making her look bad to people. But, dear me, that girl's deluded. Under the carpet? Not a chance. But I'll tell you one thing for nothing. She's always blamed him for it. Plain as day, she has. Everyone knows. It's criminal. Put all the blame on him – a 5-year-old! Can you credit it? Her own flesh and blood, too! Plain as day, like I say. She's never treated him right, ever since. It's all Carley this, Carley that – but it's like she can't stand the sight of him. She thinks no one notices, but of course everyone *does* notice. We all did, from day one. It was like she wished he was the one who was dead. So it's no wonder he's a bit wayward, is it? Bit of a rascal. Getting into trouble and that. No one to care, and that's the truth of it. No one to care.'

'And he blames himself, as well. It's so obvious.'

'Course he does, love. She's brainwashed him, that's what she's done. And you know the very worst of it? All he wants in the world is for that mother of his to love him. But you think that'll ever happen? Pigs'll fly first.'

I sat for some time after putting the phone down, just thinking. Well, not even thinking, just feeling, really – feeling my way around what I'd been told, trying to get my head round all the implications. Because, psychologically, this was huge. It also explained so much; it had obviously shaped Jenson's personality. And no wonder he'd been so keen to keep his mother's secret. She'd obviously done a pretty good job on him.

Horrible thing, guilt. Misplaced guilt, particularly. Misplaced guilt dumped on a poor innocent child, definitely. I finished my cold coffee and mentally rolled up my sleeves. I was suddenly seeing Jenson in a very different light.

Chapter 18

Jenson withdrew from me again – almost as I'd expected – but I decided to give him space. I understood why – he was probably terrified I'd start asking questions he didn't want to answer. So it was fine. I just felt so, so sorry for him. I couldn't stop thinking about how much of a load he was carrying, and how much (if what Mrs Clark had said was true, and I believed it was) he must blame, and perhaps hate, himself.

Tragically, this was all too common an occurrence. I'd fostered half a dozen kids now and dealt with many more in my previous job, and one constant with the kids with all the most challenging behaviours was self-loathing; self-esteem that went through the floor. It's not something most well-adjusted kids would even think about, but children who've been damaged emotionally by being in the care of damaged adults almost always, in my experience, felt they were to blame. Didn't matter if they'd been sexually abused, beaten, neglected or otherwise ill-treated; for all the myriad ways damaged adults could damage their children, it always ended up with one damning outcome, that the child in question felt they had somehow deserved it.

This was what dysfunctional parents did best; transferred their own issues onto the children in their care, causing the cycle to continue in perpetuity. It was a well-known fact that when abused children's problems weren't addressed, they often went on to become abusers. The kids of drug addicts, alcoholics, chaotic and neglectful parents had their life chances, day by day, month on month, year on year, gradually, inexorably eroded away. And some of those kids – a sizeable proportion, of them, probably – would go on to become dysfunctional parents themselves. That was the way it worked. That was the tragedy. Jenson was 9 now. Before too long this troubled child would become a troubled teenager. By which time – assuming he went home, and assuming his mother continued to land her guilt on him – it might be too late to get him back on the right track.

'Bloody hell, Case,' said Mike, when I found a moment to relate to him what I'd learned from Mrs Clark. 'Why on *earth* weren't we told this at the start?'

I felt dispirited having to fill Mike in on it all. They'd all bounced in from football pink cheeked and smiling. Georgie and Jenson had even had a running race home. And now I'd spoilt the mood – brought the day whomping back down to earth – as the implications of the neighbour's revelations began to sink in. Like me, Mike was hard-wired to see the bigger picture. From being a regular kind of lad in a short temporary placement, Jenson's future looked suddenly so bleak.

'I have no idea,' I said. 'I mean, it would have been a key issue, wouldn't it? So my guess is that social services don't even know. And why would they, when you think about it? She wasn't known to social services before that.'

'But she must have been, surely? Leaving a 5-year-old and a 2-year-old – and then a drowning. *Surely* they must have been aware. There'd have been an inquest, wouldn't there? Surely alarm bells must have rung.' He shook his head. 'Sheesh. It's no wonder her kids are off the rails, is it? God, what a tragedy. What a blight on the whole family. How d'you ever come to terms with something like that?'

'I doubt you ever can,' I said. 'And it gives you more of an insight into Karen, doesn't it? Not in terms of excusing her behaviour towards poor Jenson, obviously. But, well – you just can't imagine how she must feel inside, can you? However much she's not done the right thing by him – and she hasn't – she must be riddled with guilt, mustn't she? It must eat at her all the time.'

And it ate at me, on and off, for the rest of the weekend. But in some ways this was actually a positive. Knowing the child was obviously key to being able to help them, and for all that it saddened me to know what had happened, I also felt more confident that we *could* be of help to Jenson. We couldn't change the past, but we could definitely influence the future. Now his behaviour had a tangible foundation, we could set to work on it – which was exactly what I intended to do.

And Sunday night held another unexpected positive. Once I'd put the boys to bed, ironed their uniforms and helped Mike finish off clearing the tea things, I got out my laptop to catch up on my emails. I'd not been near it since the Friday, and among the usual list of spam and marketing stuff were two from social services which were of interest. The first was from a woman called Mandy, who was apparently Georgie's new social worker. Since his move from the children's home, his care plans had obviously changed, and she was going to call to arrange to meet up and discuss progress.

The other was from Marie Bateman with the excellent news that it had been decided that Jenson could have some phone contact with Karen. No, he wouldn't be able to see her till the checks on the fiancé had been completed, but this was something at least, and I knew it would really cheer him up; the first one, assuming it was all right with me, had been provisionally scheduled for Monday teatime.

'That's great, love,' said Mike, once we finally made it to the sofa. 'At least he won't feel quite so abandoned now.' He rolled his eyes and tutted. 'That's assuming she actually finds time to discuss *him*, rather than wittering on again about her flipping fiancé.'

I grabbed the remote. 'God, we're becoming a pair of old cynics, aren't we?'

Mike laughed. 'Mr and Mrs Outraged from Tunbridge Wells, that's us. And you're surprised?'

I started flicking through the channels, looking for something to watch. *Lewis*. Or *Morse*. Or *Midsomer Murders*. Nice bit of brutal murder to cheer us up. 'You know,' I said. 'I wonder what people who live in Tunbridge Wells think about it?'

'About what?' said Mike.

'About being tagged as being outraged all the time.'

'What do you think, dozy? Outraged, of course!'

It was a complete joy to be able to tell Jenson the good news about his phone call when he appeared in the kitchen for breakfast on Monday morning.

'Yesssss!' he said, jumping up and punching the air with such gusto that poor Georgie, who was just putting his empty cereal bowl in the sink, almost jumped out of his skin. So perhaps, being the bearer of good news, I'd been forgiven for interrogating him on Saturday. 'I can tell her about my game, and how I might be playing footie with Kieron's proper team next week, can't I? She'll be well proud. *Well* proud of that.'

I smiled, seeing how excited how was at this prospect. But I also felt sad. It was such a little thing, really, but clearly playing in Kieron's 'proper' team – something he'd said might be able to happen, when they'd come home from the match – was a *huge* thing for Jenson. There would be some sort of local league where he lived, I didn't doubt. But actually getting involved in such things required a modicum of parental involvement. You needed to be signed up, have a parent drop you off and pick you up. Do all the lift shares, pay the subs, procure the kit. And some parents, to be brutal about it, just couldn't be bothered.

I could see Jenson had suddenly thought of something else; his face had clouded over. 'Casey, you din't tell her anything, did you? You didn't tell her I said owt, or anything?'

'Of *course* not,' I said, shaking my head. 'I told you, I wouldn't *dream* of it. Don't you worry about that. Everything is fine.'

Which it wasn't and which it wouldn't be – not till it was brought out into the open and talked about. But that was for another day and, I guessed, ultimately, not for me to worry about. In the here and now – Jenson, reassured now, was once again smiling – it would have to do.

Just as I suspected, John knew nothing about Sammy. 'Why don't you call Marie,' he suggested, 'and see if they have anything on file. Mind you, like you, I imagine they didn't know anything about it. It's not the sort of detail that, if you *did* know, would slip your mind.'

Actually, when I got through to Marie, it seemed she did know, though like me she had only just found out. 'Isn't that funny?' she said. 'I only found out myself on Friday. And quite by chance, as well. I was just doing the final visit with Karen and Gary – tying up the paperwork and so on – when I remarked on a photo. It was one of the kids when they were younger and I wondered who the little tot was, and of course she told me. I was gobsmacked, I can tell you. Goes right through you, something like that, doesn't it?

You know, for all that she's so feckless, my heart really went out to her, poor thing.'

'I know,' I said. 'Every parent's absolute worst nightmare. And it's shed a whole new light on Jenson for me; it really explains so much. You know, she kinds of blames him? Well, that's the strong impression I get, anyway. He completely blames himself, at least, and that's got to have come from somewhere. And it would certainly explain the way she seems so down on him compared to Carley. Do you know what happened afterwards? Was there a follow-up after the inquest?'

'Apparently not,' Marie said. 'She was quite open about it. In fact, she thought we knew all about it. They didn't bring any charges. She took a stupid risk and paid the ultimate price for it. Gone no more than a few minutes, literally. Stupid, irresponsible and reprehensible – no doubt about it. But not criminal. And I imagine the thinking at the time was that this was just a tragic accident, and that she'd never be so foolish again. Let's face it, there's no punishment the courts could have inflicted that could be worse than the punishment she had already suffered.'

All of which was true, of course. But there was no escaping the fact that here we were, five years later, and she'd gone and left them again. And just a little bit further than the corner shop.

But that was something I kind of understood now. The ramifications of such a tragedy would have had far-reaching consequences. Could have been – probably *would* have been – the start of a downward spiral. Karen's family weren't unique in that respect. The death of a child affects everyone, and in lots of different ways. The siblings of dead children – their parents driven crazy by grief – often manifested all sorts of signs of emotional distress. Which led to bad behaviour, which made them challenging, which made for increasingly difficult relationships – a vicious circle that could be very hard to break. I didn't doubt this was what had happened in Jenson's case. It would always have been there between them, this terrible thing they shared. No wonder poor Jenson had freaked out at the prospect that he might be expected to look after Georgie.

Happily, my chat with Georgie's new social worker, Mandy, was more positive. She'd spent the week reading up on all his little ways and needs, and was looking forward to meeting us all the following week. As I put the phone down and prepared to start my bout of Monday housework, I reflected that, though outwardly the more challenging, Georgie was actually no trouble at all. His world – if those needs were met – was actually quite a calm place, his passage through life – provided he was placed with a family who could support him – potentially peaceful and drama-free.

Which, for the moment at least, I hoped ours would continue to be as well. But, as is always the case, no such luck.

I was on my way to Riley's when the phone rang. I'd been itching to get round there and catch up on all her news. While we'd been up to our eyes in challenging 9-year-olds, she and David had been facing their own challenges. They'd spent Saturday morning doing one of their fostering-training sessions and I couldn't wait to hear how it had gone. They were some way through the process now, and I remembered this bit of the training well. It was one of the sessions where you had to do all sorts of different role-playing, and I'd mischievously not enlightened them too much about what to expect.

Though not just out of mischief; I didn't want to stress David unduly. Because when we'd done it Mike had found it mortifying, and, had he known what was coming, he might well have ducked out. Confident as he was in his day-to-day life, he'd found the acting bit an absolute nightmare.

One scenario in particular had his toes curling so much that, had he been able to, I think he would have run for the hills. He had to play a foster dad trying to defuse a difficult situation – trying to protect himself from the full-on sexual advances of an over-amorous teenager.

He was as appalled by the very prospect, let alone the excruciating business of having to role play with an Oscar-worthy female trainer. But it was important – and little did we know quite *how* important. In just a couple of years he would find himself having to do just that with our second foster child, Sophia – one of the most challenging and tricky situations he'd yet tackled.

In truth, thinking back to that, I was now feeling very slightly guilty. Perhaps I should have prepared them after all. I'd get a ticking off from my daughter, I didn't doubt.

Except, pulling my phone out, I could see I might not get there anyway. The display showed the call was from school.

It was Andrea Cappleman. 'I imagine you're sick of hearing from me, Casey,' she said. 'But I'm afraid we've had another incident with both your boys, and I need you to come and pick Jenson up.'

'I knew it couldn't last,' I said, sighing, as I reached for my car keys. 'Go on then. What's he done to him this time?'

'To Georgie? No, no. Nothing. Far from it. No, it's a bit more complicated than that. Only just unravelled the details, but I'd be grateful if you'd just come up for Jenson. He's in a bit of a state, and there's really no point in him going back into class once lunch is done.'

It would be lunchtime right now, of course. 'No worries,' I said. 'I'll come right away.'

I should have expected it, of course. After what had happened over the weekend, Jenson was bound to be unsettled and agitated. But I was also exasperated. This kicking-off thing really needed addressing. He must surely have considered the potential consequences of his actions. He was due a contact phone call. He had football planned with Kieron for the next weekend. He had his new DS game. Had he been on our behavioural programme, all these privileges would, potentially, have been lost. That was how it worked. That was why it modified behaviour. That's how children regained control of their self-esteem. If there was one thing I should do today, I decided, as I pulled into the school driveway, it was to get Jenson with the programme, as it were.

Jenson himself was the first person I saw when I arrived in school, having been buzzed in by the school secretary. As he would be, as he was stationed on the miscreant's chair, which was right outside Andrea Cappleman's office. Her door was slightly ajar.

'You've gotta just come in with me,' he told me sullenly, as he rose from the chair. He was still crying, in an exhausted, I give up, kind of way. I thought back to the cheeky chappy we first met that day in the garden, entertaining us all with his Michael Jackson impressions; now he just looked like Hercules – a boy with the weight of the whole world on his shoulders.

Which apparently he did have. 'Now, then, Jenson,' Andrea Cappleman said, as we reconvened on two chairs in her office. 'Come on, dry your eyes and pull yourself together. We've had our chat and that's the end of it. Come on –' She plucked a tissue from the box on her desk. 'Buck up and blow your nose.'

Jenson took the proffered tissue and began scrubbing at his cheeks with it. 'So,' I asked, 'what did happen? He's been fighting again, I take it?'

'I'm afraid so,' Andrea Cappleman said. 'And, as I've made clear to Jenson, it really has to stop. We'll be breaking up for the holidays soon, and the last thing I want is to have to exclude any of my big boys from all the fun things we have planned. Eh, Jenson?'

Jenson duly nodded.

'But what about?' I said, directing the question at Jenson.

'About Jenson thinking he's a one-man vigilante band,' Andrea Cappleman said and, as Jenson wiped his eyes, she flashed me a quick smile. 'Which is something we do not have in this school.'

'Vigilante?' I asked, confused.

She nodded. 'Yes, and I absolutely understand why he feels he needs to do it. I *do*, Jenson, and I applaud your sense of right and wrong, as well. But taking matters into your own hands – and then brawling in the playground – is not the way we get our problems solved.' She turned to me. 'So we've made a pact,' she said. 'Jenson knows, don't you, that any time he sees anyone bullying Georgie, what are you to do, Jenson?'

'Tell a teacher,' Jenson mumbled.

'Exactly,' Andrea said. 'And –'

I raised my hand. 'Hang on a minute. I don't think I'm up to speed here. Who exactly has been fighting and bullying who here? I'm confused.'

She sighed. 'It's one boy in particular – the boy Jenson laid into today, of course – but to be frank with you we do have an unfortunate little gaggle of them to deal with. Year Six boys – often gets this way at this time of year. They're all ready to move on to high school – and a power of good it does them, too. To go from being king-of-the-hill now to the lowest of the low come September. But in the meantime we're having to be super-vigilant. Georgie's mostly left alone, bless him, but this particular boy seems to have it in for him.' She directed her gaze at me. 'There are, sadly, some ongoing issues ...' She trailed off, obviously not wanting to elaborate, but I knew that look – as with most bullies, there would be something at the core of it, some upset at home he was acting out about in school.

Not unlike Jenson, in fact, I thought. But I was about to hear something completely unexpected. 'And of course, Jenson,' said Andrea Cappleman, 'who is obviously Georgie's BFF and loyal protector, has been getting somewhat hot under the collar these past couple of weeks. And we have spoken about it before, and we've agreed that fighting is *never* acceptable, but today it's just all boiled over, and it has to stop.'

I could tell by her tone that she was trying to ensure she got the balance right. Yes, he needed to be disciplined, but still to know he held the moral high ground. A tricky balance, but she seemed to be managing it. I could almost see the change in Jenson's physical demeanour as she explained to me that this boy and his gang had been cruelly taunting Georgie in the dining hall, calling him a freak for only eating quiche, rice and sweetcorn every lunchtime and then, with his little gang, physically bullying him as well, pulling his hair, calling him a girl and pinching bits of sweetcorn off his plate and throwing them.

The teaching assistant, who by now had noticed something was happening, had apparently intervened and told the boys to take their trays and go and sit somewhere else. This done, and with the teaching assistant now sitting with a frightened Georgie, Jenson, infuriated, but knowing he mustn't get into trouble, had watched and waited till the boy and his crew had gone out into the playground, where, furious that they hadn't even been properly disciplined (which they hadn't, as the extent of their bullying hadn't at that point been spotted), took matters into his own hands and given the boy a proper pasting.

Naturally, the dinner lady, not knowing any of the background, had promptly dragged Jenson off to the head's office, and, as she would do, had simply reported what she'd found: that he'd set upon the boy in an unprovoked attack.

'An' that's what always happens!' Jenson protested now, suddenly more animated. 'Just like last time, and the time before, when he said he was gonna push Georgie's head in the litter bin, and like *every* time. An' I'm sick of it!' He turned to me. 'An you as well, Casey!' he threw in for good measure. 'I never told him to get those stones! Never!'

'All right, Jenson, enough of that,' said Andrea Cappleman, pushing the tissue box towards him. 'Don't start getting yourself worked up all over again. No one is blaming you today, are they? And I'm sure Casey is very proud of you for being so loyal to Georgie. But, as we've agreed, there must be no more of this fighting. It's not the way, okay?' She smiled then. 'Right. End of lecture.'

'Well,' I said as I stood up, ready to take Jenson home. 'This has all been something of an eye-opener, I must say. And I think I have an apology to make to you, Jenson. I had no idea you were looking out for Georgie so well. And Mrs

Cappleman is right. I am *very, very* proud of you. And so will Mike be, when I tell him.'

I opened my arms then, and Jenson surprised me by throwing himself into them, and as I kissed the top of his head it felt almost like I might burst, he was hugging me so tightly. Too much emotion for a Monday, I thought. Way too much emotion. 'But no more fighting, okay?' I said. 'Promise?' And Andrea Cappleman and I exchanged grins.

'Quite,' she said to Jenson. 'Now, then, tomorrow is a new day. New day, and new strategy, because I don't want to have to send you home again. Because you know what?' Jenson blinked at her. 'We *miss* you!'

'Come on then, kiddo,' I said, as I opened the car door to let Jenson jump in. 'Let's get you home and cheered up a bit. Don't forget Mum's calling at teatime and we don't want you sounding all gloomy when you talk to her, do we? She'll think I've been doing some of my ninja karate moves on you or something.'

This produced a laugh. 'Fat chance, Casey,' he said, buckling up. 'You're way too tiny to put *anyone* down, you are.'

'Oh, fighting talk is it?' I said, starting the engine. 'You'll rue saying that, my boy, and that's a promise!'

And we both laughed and joked almost all the way home, but at the same time I felt absolutely awful.

* * *

And I wasn't done with being reminded how I'd messed up with Jenson. No, it was true that I couldn't have known what had really been going on at school – *How could I? Nobody had told me!* – but I'd never been one to make excuses for myself, and I wasn't about to start now.

When the call came from Karen, just after six, as pre-arranged, I suggested Jenson go in the garden to chat to her. Mike was busy deleting the viewed *Countdown* listings on the Sky planner, Georgie just having watched one, and the boy himself had headed upstairs with his tin of precious stones. I followed him up with a basket of washing I'd just brought in off the washing line, and once I'd put it down by the airing cupboard door, ready to fold and put the towels away, I noticed Georgie humming to himself and gazing out his bedroom window.

His hair seemed to grow like wildfire – it was at least a couple of inches longer than when he'd come to us, and as I went into the room, stepping carefully over the row of stones at the entrance, I wondered how they'd dealt with it at the children's home. Did they sneak in and hack a length off while he slept?

He turned as I approached, and I was shocked when he made eye contact. 'Casey,' he said. 'We love Jenson, don't we?'

It was very, very rare for Georgie to look any of us in the eye, so I knew that this must be important.

'We do,' I agreed, as his eyes slipped away again. 'We love Jenson and we also love Georgie.'

'Jenson is a good boy. He likes green and he is a good boy,' he said, turning once again to look out of the window. 'Jenson likes green stones and Georgie likes white stones. Jenson needs a present today. Jenson isn't bad. Jenson is a *good* boy.'

I followed Georgie's gaze, and that was when it hit me. His bedroom was at the back and it looked down over the gardens. Our garden, and – God, *of course!* – our next-door neighbours' garden. Where, spread below us, was their perfectly appointed and beautifully planted rockery, with all its alpines and slabs of York stone, and neat arrays of different-coloured gravel. All those stones, laid out so neatly. So enticingly.

I had no way of knowing it for certain, but it didn't matter. It seemed so obvious now that, had I a spare leg, I would have kicked myself, hard. Jenson hadn't told Georgie to go in there. No one had. He had done it entirely by himself.

I left Georgie to it, then, and took myself off to the bathroom. I was stunned at my stupidity, stunned by my lack of insight, and staggered, *truly* staggered, that what had always seemed so natural – my ability to read kids – had so utterly deserted me in Jenson's case. I could hear him in the garden below, laughing as he talked to his mother, and the sound of patio chairs being moved – probably Mike, pottering about. And, alone with my thoughts – how on earth could I have failed him so badly? – I sat down on the edge of the bath and cried.

Chapter 19

I felt so much better when I woke up the next morning. Better and also energised. Having redefined my role in supporting both Georgie and Jenson, everything suddenly seemed so much easier. It was mad, really, I thought, how the mind worked. All the time I had convinced myself Jenson was one type of child, I had only allowed myself to work with him in a certain way. A simple shift in focus and it was as if the world had opened up again, and I could only now begin to see the big picture. It had been a tough lesson to take on board, and one I was determined not to forget.

The rest of the week passed without incident. And not least because the change in Jenson was palpable. No words were said; we discussed neither the death of his little sister nor his feelings about what happened (that was something I knew I shouldn't force) but it was as if he could tell I felt differently about him; that I understood him better, which was true.

I was therefore looking forward to the following week-end. The forecast was glorious, both weather-wise and home-wise – free from the permanent undercurrent of anxiety about having to be braced for potential flashpoints between the boys.

But they were going to be there whether I was braced for them or not, as, on Saturday morning, I was about to find out.

'Mum?' said Riley, calling me first thing that morning. 'Get the kettle on. I'm on my way over with Jackson. David's taken Levi to his dad's to do something manly like fixing cars, so I thought I'd come to yours a little earlier.'

I got the coffee on and mugs out, smiling as I did so. There was no day, however lovely, that couldn't be made lovelier by the addition of my daughter and little grandson. And today did look like being a lovely one, definitely. Mike had gone into work for a couple of hours, and as soon as he was back he'd promised the boys he'd take the pair of them to watch Kieron play football, and perhaps have a knock around themselves, while I went into town with Riley and Jackson. Jenson was particularly excited about seeing Kieron, I knew, because only the other evening he'd told him he was a brilliant footballer and that there might be a chance for him to join the junior team.

He came clattering into the kitchen now – clattering being the operative word: he was already suited and booted for football, right down to the new football boots Mike had bought for him.

'My, you're keen, love,' I said, laughing. 'Mike won't be back for another hour yet!'

'Does it look good, Casey?' he wanted to know, grinning as he struck a pose for me, then throwing in a short moon-walk for good measure. Which was good to see, but not that good, I decided, remembering the boots, which were studded.

'A lot better than my kitchen floor's going to look, matey, once you've finished scraping those studs across it!' I scolded. But I was still smiling. When he was being like this, smiling became infectious. 'You know what you look like?' I told him. 'A mini Kenny Dalglish.'

'Kenny what? Who the hell's he?'

'Less of the "hell", love, if you don't mind! He's a famous footballer. Played for Liverpool, back in ...' I shook my head, seeing Jenson's blank expression. 'Oh, never mind. I'm getting old. You won't have heard of him. Hi, sweetie,' I added, seeing Georgie come in as well. 'You all right?'

Georgie pointed to the cup cupboard.

'Are you thirsty? I asked him, saying the words slowly. I was on something of a mission to get him to actually ask for the things he wanted. He certainly had enough vocabulary. I was sure he just pointed to pictures because that was what he'd got used to doing, both in school and obviously in the children's home.

He nodded. 'Georgie is thirsty,' he agreed. 'Milk please.'

'Good boy,' I said, filling up a beaker with milk. 'So, what do you think of Jenson today, eh?'

Georgie glanced at Jenson, who was once again posing in his footie kit.

'Jenson is a good boy,' Georgie said at length. 'And Jenson has very shiny hair today.'

I laughed as Jenson, also giggling, ran his hand through his mop of hair, as if modelling in an advert for shampoo. Then he gestured to the back door. 'You wanna come outside,' he asked Georgie, 'and kick my ball around with me?' And to my slight surprise Georgie smiled at him and nodded.

I watched them play for a few minutes, listening to them through the open patio door, and being amused, as Jenson tried to explain the business of tackling other players, and how as long as you were going for the ball and not the person it was completely acceptable to knock people over. Jenson understood now, as well as Mike and I did, that you had to be careful about the words you used with Georgie as, because of his autism, he took everything so literally. Only a couple of days earlier we'd had the makings of a proper scream-fest, just because Jenson had told us a joke in the car on the way home from school. It wasn't the joke itself; it was the fact that he finished up by saying that when he told it to Mike later he'd 'probably laugh his head off'.

It never crossed my mind but, of course, this had been playing on Georgie's mind ever since, and when Jenson repeated the joke over tea, and Mike duly started laughing, Georgie clamped his hands over his ears and promptly burst into tears.

It had taken a while for any of us to work out what was wrong with him. It was only when he kept pointing to Mike and whimpering that the penny finally dropped. And once it had, and we'd gently probed the cause of his distress, he managed to explain that he was really expecting Mike's head to fall off.

I tried hard over the next few days to explain such figures of speech to Georgie. I tried to explain how when you said when you were so hungry you could eat a horse you didn't actually plan to eat one – you'd just have your tea. I tried to explain that when people said it was raining cats and dogs it didn't actually mean the sky was full of animals, just that the rain was so heavy it felt like it must be something more than just drops of water. But the more examples I tried to come up with, the more ridiculous and illogical it all seemed – even to me! How on earth did our language become so bizarre? And if it felt that way to me, how must it feel to someone like Georgie, whose use of language was so concrete and literal? The world and the people in it must feel like such a strange and scary place to him. And though I got precisely nowhere in my quest to get him to see beyond the literal, in looking at things through his eyes I learned something at least. And I was soon to have a rather more graphic illustration of how simple was Georgie's way of seeing things.

When Riley arrived, minutes later, she climbed out of the taxi and signalled that she wanted me to come out and give her a hand. She had Jackson in her arms and needed me to help her get the buggy out of the boot, and then put it up so she could lay Jackson down in it.

'Oh, my –' I began.

'Shh,' she said, putting finger to her lips as I approached her. 'He's only just gone off,' she explained, once I'd put the buggy up so she could lay him down. 'He didn't have the best of nights last night, and he's been a right grump since he was up. He'll be in a much better mood once he's had an hour of kip, I'm sure. And so will I,' she added, grimacing. 'So will I.'

The taxi driver paid, she pushed the buggy down the path and I followed. 'I was going to say,' I began again, 'that your hair looks … erm … nice.' Though the more accurate word might have been 'arresting'. She'd dyed it – in fact, presumably bleached it, then dyed it – so that, rather than her usual raven black, same as mine was, it was now a show-stopping shade of flame red.

She turned and pulled a face as she tipped the front of the buggy up over the doorstep, then gently parked a sleeping Jackson in the hallway.

'Cheers,' she said, grinning. 'Thanks for the compliment, Mum. I don't think!'

'I do like it,' I rushed to reassure her. 'It was just a bit of shock, that's all. I'm sure I'll get used to it. Are you pleased with it? It certainly looks nice and shiny.'

'I *love* it,' she said. 'I just get sick of being so dark all the time. I fancied a change.' She smoothed it down. 'So I went and got one.'

I was just about to agree – because, in fact, I was already getting used to it – when Georgie appeared in the hallway, flushed from his bout of Jenson-style football training. And I was just about to ask him how it had gone when I realised he was beginning to be distressed about something – he had flattened himself against the far wall in the hallway and was rigid, staring fixedly at the ceiling.

'You all right, love?' I asked him, confused about what was wrong with him. 'Look, here's Jackson, come to see us. He's just having a little sleep, then he'll probably want a play with you. I'll get the bricks out in a bit so you can build him one of your towers, eh?'

Georgie, quite naturally, I supposed, loved building towers. He would arrange bricks and blocks with such precision that you could take a spirit level to them, and no angle would be anything less than perfect. And, strangely – he was such a conundrum, in so many ways – he didn't seem to mind that the little ones would then send his creations skittering all over the floor. He'd just gather them up, one by one, into little piles, and stack them up all over again.

But he didn't seem interested, and I suddenly realised my mistake. What had I been thinking? I should have told him that Riley was on her way over. What a klutz! If I'd done that one simple thing he wouldn't be in the tizz he was now. That was all that had been needed, that simple bit of preparation, so that Riley's arrival didn't come out of the blue.

I motioned to Riley to go into the kitchen and, as she walked past him, I noticed Georgie visibly wince. 'It's all right, love,' I reassured him. 'I should have told you they were coming, shouldn't I? But we're going into the kitchen now. Why don't you go back into the garden with Jenson and play, eh? Or into the living room, perhaps. Shall I put *Countdown* on for you?'

Neither option seemed to appeal – he shook his head violently at both suggestions – so, in the end, I decided it would be best if I just got out of his face. He didn't look close to having a full-on freak-out or anything – just unsettled by this unexpected event happening in his day. If I left him for five minutes I felt sure that he'd calm down. He just needed to get back on track again. He did accept a gentle hand steering him into the living room, at least, so that's where I left him, safe on the sofa, waiting for the security of Mike's return and the trip to football.

'He must be a handful at times,' Riley observed quietly, once I joined her in the kitchen. 'But I guess at the same time you must be learning such a lot.'

'Something new every day,' I agreed. 'Literally, every day. Because there's no one definitive set of "rules" with autism spectrum disorders. Every child is so incredibly different, and complex.' And I was just in the middle of elaborating for Riley – explaining the reasons for Georgie's discomfort on seeing them – when I was interrupted by the sound of a cry.

'You hear that?' Riley said.

I nodded. 'It sounded like Jackson.' But at the same time it sounded odd. We both went and put our heads around the kitchen door.

It took a moment, since the buggy had been parked facing away from us, but just as the pair of us realised it was empty the act was confirmed by another cry – coming from upstairs. And then more of a scream. It *was* Jackson. We both looked automatically towards the stairwell, and then, putting two and two together, towards the now empty living room, before thundering, almost as one, up the stairs.

'What's going on?' Jenson wanted to know, now clattering up behind us, having obviously heard Jackson's cries as well.

'Oh my God,' Riley was saying. 'What's he done with him? God, if he's hurt him ...'

My heart leapt into my mouth. We had previous in that regard, and I was all too aware of it. Previous foster kids who'd given us similar scares with the little ones. So what had possessed me to think it would be perfectly okay to leave Jackson in his buggy in the hall with Georgie close by and so obviously stressed? What had I been *thinking*?

An unpalatable image rose, unbidden, into my mind. Of that day, early on, when Georgie had attacked Jenson. Oh, God. But he couldn't. Surely he wouldn't – why on earth would he want to hurt Jackson? And more to the point, I thought, as we ran into his bedroom, scattering half his entrance stones, where the hell was Jackson? Where had Georgie taken him?

It had only been a matter of minutes since we'd left them. No more than that – and we'd only been a few feet away. Yet where was he now? All we could see was Georgie, sitting cross-legged on his bed, hugging his collection tin close to his chest and rocking violently.

I could tell Riley was struggling to keep her composure, yet she still did an admirable job. 'Georgie,' she said softly. 'Where's baby Jackson? Where's the baby gone, sweetheart? Can you tell me?'

Georgie flinched with every word she spoke to him, his teeth clenching, and I realised we were heading towards that freak-out after all.

I stepped closer, and was just about to try to speak to him myself when we all heard a soft but distinct whimpering. And it took less than a second to work out where it was coming from.

'The wardrobe!' Riley exclaimed. 'He's shut Jackson in the wardrobe! Oh, God …' She rushed across to yank it open.

Except she couldn't. And it didn't take a brain surgeon to realise why. He'd locked the door and taken the key out.

Once again I berated myself. The key! The bloody door key! Why hadn't I thought to remove the door key when we moved Georgie in there?

'Georgie,' I said, trying to keep my voice calm and level, as Jackson's whimpers began increasing in pitch and volume. 'Where's the key, love? You need to tell me where the key to the wardrobe door is …'

Riley was still trying to force the door, increasingly anxiously. 'It's okay, baby,' she tried to soothe a clearly terrified Jackson. 'It's okay, baby. Mummy's just got to get the key. Everything's okay … Georgie!' she barked then, turning to him. 'You *must* tell us where the key is! We have to get Jackson out. Can't you hear him? *Listen*. See? He's terrified!'

But Georgie could hear nothing. That much was obvious. All he could do was rock and, once again, seeing Riley, flinch and cower. Which made no sense to me at all. Where had this all *come* from?

But there was someone in the room with us who'd clearly seen something I hadn't. Jenson, who I had almost forgotten was even standing there, now stepped past me and sat down on the bed beside Georgie. Not too close – not so close that it might traumatise Georgie further – but certainly close enough to get his attention.

'Georgie, mate,' he said, pointing to my, by now, almost crying daughter. 'You are *so* clever, mate. You really are. Good boy,' he added. 'Georgie's done *good* here. Good boy for protecting Riley's baby.'

I couldn't quite make sense of what I was hearing, and I could see Riley hadn't either. Where was this coming from? But Jenson was too busy to even notice my confused expression. All his attention was focused on Georgie, as well as his gaze, which was encouraging and direct. 'Good boy,' he said again, and now he did glance in my direction. 'Good boy, because you're spot on. It *could* have been a stranger. Except it's not.' He risked a light touch on Georgie's arm. He didn't flinch from it. 'It *could* have been a stranger, but actually it *is* Riley. She's just got some weird-coloured paint stuff in her hair. Which makes it red. But it's still Riley, *honest* it is, mate. But you were good, 'cos if it *were* a stranger you would have saved the baby. That's right, isn't it, Casey? He would have saved Jackson, wouldn't he?'

I nodded firmly, still too stunned to speak.

'So now we need the key, okay?' he finished. He gestured to Georgie's tin. 'You got it in there?'

I was gobsmacked. Which, with the things I've seen, is not something that happens to me that often. Our little hero! Where on earth had he developed the insight to work that out so cleverly?

'Have you, Georgie?' I asked him. 'Is it in there? Is it in your tin?'

Georgie didn't respond directly, but he did move his hands across the tin lid for a few seconds. Then, finally, at Jenson's gentle prompting, he removed it. He then pulled out the heavy antique key, complete with tassel, and, after staring at her hard, he passed Riley the key.

'Clever boy, Georgie,' she said, cottoning on, and taking possession of it, upon which one very fractious toddler was finally released. 'Oh, you clever boy, Jenson!' Riley said, as she scooped Jackson up from the pile of old bedding he'd been sitting on. 'If my hands weren't already full, there'd be no escape from my clutches, believe me. I'd be giving you *such* an enormous bear hug right now.'

And though Jenson's expression was suitably 9-year-old-boy horrified at that prospect, we could both see just how much he glowed with pride.

'Blimey. You live and learn, don't you?' said Mike, once he returned from work, half an hour later, and Riley and I had filled him in on the latest drama. Georgie, completely fine now, was back in the living room, watching an episode of *Countdown*, while he waited to be taken to football, while a beaming Jenson took centre stage at the kitchen table.

'How on earth did you work it out, lad?' Mike asked him. 'That's some clever thinking!'

'I was just remembering what I'd heard Casey saying about how Georgie understood meanings,' he told him. 'An' about his pictures. How he looked at things to know what they were. An' the hair. I remembered when me mum had her hair bleached once. And when I come home from school, and she was standing in the garden with our Carley – an' how I didn't recognize her – I really thought she were someone else.' He shrugged modestly. 'I just thought of all that, really.'

'Well, you thought brilliantly,' Riley said. '*Brilliantly*. So you should give yourself a medal – even if you *did* call it weird-coloured paint stuff – because I would never have thought of that in a million trillion years.'

And she was right. And I was so pleased for him. So pleased to see him feeling so loved and valued. But it was bittersweet, because it also served to remind me of his reality. In his world, his own family – the world he would soon be going back to – that was so obviously, so painfully, not the case.

Chapter 20

The day of Riley's red hair (or, rather, as it would always be known, her 'weird-coloured paint stuff') turned out to be something of a red-letter day for all of us, because it marked a turning point – one that we only really noticed as such in hindsight – after which everything seemed to be so different.

And different in a good way. The last couple of weeks of term seemed to fly by, certainly. There were no bust-ups, no arguments, no incidents – either in school or out of it – and like the days, which were uniformly warm, dry and sunny, life trundled on entirely without drama. There was still the business of not knowing when Jenson might be returning home, of course, but with his twice-weekly phone calls from his mum to keep him going, even Jenson stopped asking when he might be heading back to her, and in one particularly fanciful moment I wondered if perhaps he felt more settled with his lot, to the extent that he was actually quite happy. He was missing his mum and sister, of course – something would have been badly amiss if he wasn't – but kids in boarding schools coped with prolonged absence from family, didn't they? And in America kids Jenson's age were packed off to summer camp for weeks on end. So was Jenson seeing it like that, perhaps? Like some sort of extended holiday?

He certainly seemed to be feeling at home now. Which was just as well, I supposed, because just a week into the start of the summer holidays I had a call from Marie to let me know that the latest child-protection conference about Karen had been cancelled. This would have been the one in which a final decision was made about both the kids returning home, but Karen herself had cancelled it at the last minute. Perhaps fearing she might not get them back, or perhaps because she was genuinely uncertain, she had told social services that she was in two minds about Gary continuing to live with them, as she wasn't 100 per cent sure she would eventually be marrying him. This naturally changed her circumstances radically – and for the better. But until she decided one way or another – including telling him to leave, if that was her decision – no decision could be made about the kids.

Although this all sounded very noble, assuming her motivation was genuine, which was what I wanted to believe, I still couldn't shift my doubts about her. What if she was just stalling because she was enjoying a bit of freedom from the burdens of motherhood? It felt cynical to think it but I couldn't get past the knowledge that the kids were now being burdened – as if they hadn't been burdened enough already – with the knowledge that she wasn't exactly fighting to get them back with her.

And Jenson did feel it, I was sure of it. 'What if someone tried to take me away from you and Mike, Casey?' he asked me one evening, after tea. 'You'd fight like a ninja to keep hold of me, wouldn't you?'

'Too right,' I said, joking that I'd do my extra-special karate kick on anyone who dared try it. But it wasn't a joke, was it? He badly needed to know that he was worth fight-ing *for*.

And then there was good news, the following Thursday. Not news about Karen, but certainly news that would take Jenson's mind off it. Mike came home from work that night clutching a bottle of red wine, and brought it into the living room after dinner, with a couple of glasses.

'So what's the occasion?' I asked him, bemused. We weren't really big on the drinking at home thing, and only on special days would we crack open the vino. Plus this was a Thursday. Which would be followed by a busy Friday.

'I have a bit of a nice surprise,' he said, pouring. 'Well, I'm hoping you'll think it's a nice surprise, anyway. Remember when we borrowed my boss's caravan for that holiday?'

Of course I did. It had been an unforgettable holiday. We'd taken Ashton and Olivia, kids we'd had who'd had the most heartbreaking start to their young lives imagina-ble. That they had never seen the sea, never felt sand between their toes, never built sandcastles or gone rock pooling could only hint at the sort of barren lives they'd endured. It was also memorable because it had been there that Ashton had finally disclosed to me the extent of the horrible abuse he'd suffered.

'We-ell,' Mike continued. 'How d'you fancy heading back there? He's given me the keys, and –'

'Given you the keys? For when?'

'For next week. Because I have the *whole of next week off!*'

'What?' I said, wide eyed. 'How on earth did you manage that?'

'Because there's a big job coming up in September and I promised I'd do lots of overtime, and because the forecast is brilliant, and because I told him I know where the bodies are buried and ... well, because he just thinks I'm wonderful, I suppose.' He chuckled. 'But mostly because we were chatting about the kids and he said it was free next week, and it's fairly quiet at work, and I have a lot of holiday to use up before the year end ...'

I put the glass down that he'd passed me while he'd been telling me all this and threw my arms around him. 'You know what?' I said. 'I think I'll have to marry you.'

So that was that. And I was thrilled, because I hadn't been expecting a holiday. We couldn't plan anything while we had everything so up in the air, and I'd contented myself with a few days in the sun once we had a couple of weeks without any kids in; as was mostly the case, going abroad with foster kids was often a no-no, simply because these kids rarely had passports.

But with things as they were, who knew when that might happen anyway? So this was a gift. An absolute gift. Though we couldn't simply pack our bags and head off on the Saturday morning. I had to figure Georgie into my thinking, and how he'd cope. I even panicked a little, once I thought about it. Could we even, in fact, go? Would he be able to cope with going away on holiday? Our Kieron had grown less and less enamoured of holidays as he'd got older, and once he was an older teenager he'd elect to have my mum and dad come and house-sit alongside him – he just hated being parted from all his routines and his things.

But speaking to Sylvia from his old children's home provided reassurance on that point.

'Oh, no, that's fine,' she reassured me, when I called her on the Friday morning. 'He's been on lots of holidays. Somewhere among his things are all his photo albums – I remember packing them. You'll find them in one of the cardboard boxes.'

Which wouldn't be difficult. There were just the two of them, Georgie not much doing possessions, bar whatever his current obsession was – in this case stones.

'Get them out and go through them with him,' she counselled. 'There are all sorts of pictures of him: on the beach, at the funfair, eating ice cream. Just go through them and explain that you'll be doing similar things.'

And it worked a treat. I sat him down with the pictures and explained we were going on holiday, and I was amazed at how quickly he got the idea. 'Georgie and Jenson and Casey and Mike going on holiday. Not Sylvia, not Franklyn, not Jenny and not Alistair. Georgie and Jenson and Casey and Mike.' He kept chanting it to himself all day.

Jenson, on the other hand, had never been on holiday. He'd been on days out at the beach and visited a holiday park a friend was staying at, but had never in his life stayed even overnight at anywhere seasidey, and I felt a real pang of anger, thinking of his mum swanning around the Med with her boyfriend and leaving her kids home alone.

But as usual Jenson's grin drove the bad thoughts from my head. He was beside himself. He really was beyond excited.

'Will Simon Cowell be there?' he wanted to know. ''Cos if he is I'll show him my moonwalk. Oh my God. I could be on *Britain's Got Talent!*'

Which had me bursting out laughing, as well as being confused. 'Why on earth would Simon Cowell be there?' I spluttered, as he pirouetted round the kitchen, practising his routine. 'What in heaven makes you think he'd turn up there?'

Logic, it seemed. Well, an illogical kind of logic. He'd seen *The X Factor*, and seen the bit where the acts went to the judges' houses, and for some reason he had got it into his head that Simon Cowell's beach house was part of a holiday park.

'An it's in Wales,' he said, with the confidence of a boy who had his facts straight.

'Barbados,' I corrected. 'I think his beach house is in Barbados.'

'I *know* it is,' he said, tutting. 'Which is in *Wales*.'

But there was scant time to get out the atlas and give Jenson a geography lesson, as, the boys primed and the washing done, it was a case of get packing, and after an early start – and a backtrack to return home for some all-important stone that had been forgotten – we arrived at the holiday park just after lunchtime that Saturday.

And as we explored the park and its facilities, a hunch I'd harboured turned out to be true. Just as I'd thought I'd remembered from our last visit there, it seemed Jenson might have his chance to show off his moonwalk after all, if not to the man himself, at least to his fellow holidaymakers.

'Look,' Mike explained, as we showed the boys the club house, 'this is where we'll probably come most evenings. They have a mini disco every night for the youngsters and a different entertainer every evening.' I was already liking the sound of it myself. A whole week away from routine and telly and the same old same old, plus sun, sea and sand, and entertainment on tap. Bliss.

'Oh, and look at this, Jenson,' Mike then said, pointing to a poster.

Can you sing like Rihanna? it asked. *Can you dance like Michael Jackson? If so, we want to see you at the Hippo's Den, on Thursday at 5 p.m. Junior talent-show rehearsal – acts to perform Friday at 6 p.m. Guest judges and great prizes to be won!*

'You see?' said Jenson, punching the air. 'It *might* be Simon Cowell coming!'

'I don't know about that,' I replied, laughing. 'But they must have known *you* were coming. Who'd have thought they'd be looking for Michael Jackson impersonators?'

'Love,' said Mike, 'have you ever been to a holiday camp, here or in fact anywhere, where they *haven't* had a Michael Jackson something going on?'

'But I'll need some music and a hat!' Jenson said, realising his key props were non-negotiable.

'Don't worry, mate,' Mike reassured him. 'I'm sure they'll be able to provide a backing track. And when we pop into Swansea to pick up some bits and bobs later, I promise we'll track you down a trilby.'

Which, after a couple of days of relaxing, going to the beach and eating ice cream, was exactly what we did. The campsite was much busier than we remembered it, but that was probably to be expected. We were in the thick of the school holidays and everyone seemed of the same mind as we – wanted to enjoy the best of the weather before the summer was over and done with and it was time to start buying pencil cases and school uniforms.

And I was pleased to see that Georgie, too, seemed to be having a good time. Though it was obvious from the outset that Jenson would be in his element, the sheer number of people and the massive amount of noise and activity all around us could, I knew, pose a major problem.

But it seemed it was sound that had the most potential for causing distress to him, as I realised when I found him one day, sitting, rocking, with his hands clamped tightly over his ears, on a garden chair that he'd parked round the back of the caravan.

I was about to ask him what was wrong when I checked myself. Perhaps I should try and imagine what it might be myself. And as I watched and listened, it slowly became apparent. I could hear what sounded like a young Elvis impersonator practising coming from the open door of the club house, I could hear shrieks coming from the swimming pool, and regular loud splashes, I could hear shouts form the adventure playground and bursts of unrestrained laughter – all the noises you'd expect to hear when children were having fun. All perfectly normal, of course, but also such an assault to Georgie's senses. It was then that I remembered something I'd read about children with autism, and how sound – certain sounds – could be extremely painful for them.

Feeling once again guilty for not having remembered it earlier, I gently encouraged Georgie to go back inside the caravan, shut the doors and windows and switched on the fan. He immediately relaxed then, and reached for a box of dominoes to play with, preferring, as ever, to do something solitary.

Mike at this time had taken Jenson swimming. In fact, it was the third time this week. It was obviously too noisy for Georgie and far too busy, but when Jenson had explained to us that he'd never been taught to swim it became Mike's major mission for the week to rectify that situation, and have him managing a width by the end of the week.

And it had turned out to be an illuminating business. After the second lesson, Mike had explained to me the previous night, once the boys were in bed, Jenson had got himself into a right state. Embarrassed at being the only 9-year-old with armbands, he'd kept insisting that he could swim without them, and, frustrated to keep failing, had stomped off and said he didn't want to learn any more.

Calming him down with the offer of a glass of pop and a pizza, Mike had sat him down and explained that, just as you couldn't run before you could walk, you had to learn in stages, which took time. At this, Jenson had promptly burst into tears, and though he obviously found it hard to articulate exactly why it made him feel as he did, he was finding it hard because it made him think of how his little sister died, and though he wasn't exactly afraid of the water – that much was obvious – it was as if somehow he was going against his mum by even learning, because she told him he must never go swimming.

'God,' Mike had said to me, 'it's so complicated, isn't it? And he must have thought we were trying to make him face his fears or something. Poor lad. It had never even occurred to me.'

We'd both agreed, though, that it was still something he should pursue. As long as Jenson was willing to stick at it, they should keep pushing on, because in doing so he was facing his fears, which was no bad thing, as well as strengthening the bond he and Mike had developed. What with the football and now the swimming they had really grown close, and making attachments (this attachment, and any positive attachment, for that matter) could only be a good thing for a latchkey kid like Jenson. These were things that would stand him in good psychological stead longer after he was no longer with us.

But it was the talent show that was Jenson's major preoccupation, and by Thursday afternoon you really would have thought he had ants in his pants, he was hopping round so much with impatience. As promised, Mike had found him a very fine hat. Encrusted with black glitter, which seemed to get everywhere in the caravan, it was the perfect trilby shape, à la Michael Jackson. He had perfected his routine – which he was doing to *Billie Jean* – right down to the very last thrust. And it was very good. I was almost as excited as he was.

'Nooo, Casey!' he said, when I suggested I might accompany him to his rehearsal. 'You can't show me up. Mums and dads don't come!' He turned to Georgie. 'You can come,' he said. 'But you and Mike can't, Casey. You'll have to stay in the clubhouse and wait to see it till tomorrow.'

So that was us told. And, of course, we wouldn't dream of 'showing him up'. I was even tickled to be bracketed in the mums and dads category, and pleased that we'd been able to quietly put him in a position where he had to temper our enthusiasm for being there. To tell mums and dads they couldn't come, you had to first be in a position where they were desperate to see you perform, after all. Which for some kids – Jenson among them, I didn't doubt – wasn't a feeling they had the luxury of often.

And I was pleased when Georgie nodded his agreement to Jenson's plan. And as the Hippo's Den was a room off the club house, and could be entered only via it, I didn't have to stress, as long as we found ourselves seats close to the main entrance, about him getting agitated and wandering off unnoticed.

Or so we thought. With two coffees and a chance of a bit of peace and quiet, in a now relatively child-free club house, we were so busy enjoying some us time that the time seemed to fly by. My main concern, given the large number of kids seeming to be involved, was that Jenson would be crushingly disappointed if he didn't win.

Mike disagreed. 'You know, I think he'll be fine with it,' he said. 'I don't think he'll care where he's placed in the competition, just as long as he gets his moment in the spotlight and a big cheer for doing it. He just needs the adulation, that kid.'

Even so, I couldn't help cross my fingers that he would storm the place, that he would be the best and that he would get that coveted first prize. I was still locked into my typical stage-school mummy thinking (picturing Jenson taking the winning bow, to massed cheers of approval) when I was disturbed from my thoughts by a young girl, tugging at my sleeve. This was a girl I recognised called Ruby, who'd palled up with Jenson and was staying in the caravan opposite ours.

'Casey,' she was saying. 'You have to come quick. It's Georgie. He's stuck on the roof and he might die!' She was obviously quite distressed.

'The *roof*?' I answered, as shocked as she was frightened. 'What roof? How on earth did he get up onto a roof?'

Mike got up, as confused as I was about how Georgie could have slipped past us. But it seemed he hadn't. We'd been wrong about there only being one exit to the Hippo's Den. There was also a fire door at the back which, though ordinarily closed, obviously, someone had decided, due to the heat generated by such a big crowd of excited performers, to open up, to let a bit of air in.

And what had happened, as Ruby explained as we followed her in and out of the fire door, was that Jenson had apparently decided – for reasons that seemed entirely in keeping with the little scamp – to climb onto the roof of the shower block, just adjacent to the building, and do an impromptu extra performance to the small crowd of kids below.

Not that he was up there right now. No, that was Georgie. He looked absolutely terrified, and was groaning as well as rocking, while just below him, standing on the small wall that was adjacent to the block, teetered Jenson, obviously trying to coax him down.

'Jenson, what's going on?' I wanted to know, while Mike started to climb up to the roof, using the route that he'd presumably used, via the wall and one of the toilet cubicle windows.

'Oh Casey, I'm so sorry!' Jenson said immediately. 'It's my entire fault he went up there. I just wanted to climb up and do my dance for everyone, and he just followed me. I didn't tell him to. I just turned round and there he was!'

'To do your dance?' I spluttered. 'To do your dance up on a roof? Jenson, are you stark staring mad?'

'I'm sorry,' he said again. 'I'm really *really* sorry. I jus' didn't think. I – I just never thought he'd follow me. Why would he *do* that?'

'Sweetheart,' I said, exasperated. 'That is not the point at all! This isn't just about Georgie – it's about you! You might have fallen and hurt yourself too! What were you thinking?'

'I don't know,' he mumbled. 'I just … I just …'

'Wanted to show off,' I said, fixing my gaze on him and frowning. 'Which could very nearly,' I added, watching with relief as Mike had hold of Georgie, 'have ended up with a nasty accident, couldn't it?'

To which Jenson had the good grace to blush.

Mike had by now got hold of Georgie and carefully helped him down to me. And as I took his arm I was at least grateful, given the small crowd around us, that Georgie seemed so stunned now that he didn't even seem to think of freaking out.

That being the case, and the shower block having been a comparatively low building, and with Jenson being – for once – so completely apologetic and contrite, once I'd reassured a traumatised campsite rep (who'd been in the toilet when it had happened), I decided I would take my mother's least-said-soonest-mended attitude, and say nothing further about the incident. Jenson had had a fright, and that had been enough to teach him a lesson. And he had also apologised, which spoke volumes about his progress.

Though I should have probably felt more disapproving than I actually did about the swelling band of fans he'd got as a result of it.

'Yo, Jenson,' said one, as we headed back to the club house later, 'you da boss!'

Jenson was already half way through his joyous air punch before he thought better of it.

Every foster kid is special, and we have cherished memories of every one of them that will stay with us, but that Friday-night talent show – starring our mini Michael Jackson – is definitely high up in my personal top ten.

Jenson wasn't ours, but I don't think either of us could have been more proud-parent excited, when, having given a faultless performance, he bounded back to sit with us to await the verdict from the pretty young compère.

'And in third place …' she called out. Not Jenson. He screwed his eyes up. 'And in second place …' Not Jenson. He clamped his hands over his eyes.

'And in first place …' I don't think any of us breathed at that point, including Georgie. 'It's our very own Tarzan …' We shrieked so loud at that point that she had to shout his name over us.

The cheer that went up then really couldn't have been more gratifying, and the applause was as sincere as it was deafening. And boy, did it go on. It continued right through him leaping up to go and collect his prize, right through his moonwalk across the stage to be presented with it, and right through his return, triumphant and beaming, bearing his certificate and ten-pound voucher to spend in the shop.

It was still ringing in my ears as he sat down beside us and then thought better of it, stood up again and threw his arms around us for a group hug. And Georgie let him. I was a complete blubbering wreck.

Chapter 21

I had half-expected to return home from holiday to an email or message from Marie Bateman or John, telling me that there'd been progress on the situation with Karen. But there was nothing, and as the days passed I became increasingly concerned, as John had promised me everything would be sorted by the start of the new term. And, more importantly, this was what Jenson had expected too. So it wasn't surprising that he was beginning to get itchy feet. He'd not physically seen his mum and sister for some weeks now.

'What's she playing at, Casey?' he asked me one day. 'I told her about my stifficate and that I'd bought her a photo frame out of my voucher money, an' she swore it would only be a few days before I'd be moving back home.'

At least the telephone contacts had continued twice weekly and, as far as I knew, had been going really well. But I so felt for him. Since we'd come back, and he'd been so full of pride, every day had chipped away at him a little more. We'd all felt a bit flat – you always tended to after a good holiday – but for Jenson it really was a dispiriting whump back to earth. Handily, however, I had called Marie for an update, and knew that the new child-protection hearing would be any day now. Perhaps then we *would* have news – positive news, fingers crossed – as it seemed Karen had decided to give 'love of my life' Gary the heave-ho. But with her clearly so fickle in matters of the heart, I didn't dare tempt fate by offering Jenson any false hope.

'I'm sure it's all happening behind the scenes, sweetie,' I assured him. 'These things all have to be done properly.'

'But *what* things have to be done?' he bleated. 'What do they have to do? Mum's said she's sorry an' she won't do it again. So what do they have to do?'

Put like that, I was hard pressed for an answer.

And I understood his impatience. I'd have been the same myself. So I tried to keep him busy with lots of activities, of which swimming, now he'd mastered the basics of doggy paddle, seemed the most important of the lot. It would be so good, I reasoned, to send him home having acquired a new skill that he could feel proud of. And I made a mental note to remind Marie about the issues around him learn-ing. If Karen was going to have the support of a regular social worker, one of the things they could begin to tackle was the tension in the relationship between Jenson and his mother. It was probably too optimistic to hope that she might begin to take him swimming herself, but him doing so might at least open up a line of communication – get her to try and face her fears as well.

In the meantime, I wanted to capitalise on Mike's work down in Wales by taking him as frequently as possible. And he was keen – so much so that when the following Saturday came round, and I mentioned that I was going to the pool with Riley and the little ones, he even chose to join us over football.

'But tell Kieron I'm sorry, an' it's only for one week,' he instructed Mike. 'It's just that now that I don't need my armbands I have to keep practising till I can do a full length. Then next term in school I can get my first stifficate.' He thought for a moment before adding, with a grin, 'An' tell him I'm getting my legs stronger an' all for footy, so it's all good. I'll be even *better*.'

Jenson was even happier when I told him that the plan was that we'd all be going to a café for hot dogs and ice creams afterwards.

And we had a fine time, as you tend to when you know the result of your labours would be a trio of tired and happy children. After a fun hour and a half in the pool, I left the car in the pool car park and we all had a stroll into town for lunch.

It was one of those cafés where they had an area sectioned off for children, so after getting Jenson and Levi settled at a table with colouring books and pencils I eventually sat down with Riley and Jackson, who had fallen fast asleep in his buggy. It was only then I noticed I had a missed call on my mobile.

'Oh shit!' I said to Riley. 'John Fulshaw's been trying to reach me. I wonder what he wants on a Saturday.' And I *did* wonder. John would only call at the weekend if it was something that required either his or my attention.

'Phone him back then,' Riley said, obviously seeing the concerned look on my face. 'The boys are otherwise occupied. I'll keep an eye on things. Go on.'

I took myself and my phone out into the street and pressed ring back. Would this be news about Jenson, or Georgie, or both?

'Oh hi, Casey,' he said, answering almost immediately. 'Thanks for getting back to me so quickly. I thought I'd better ring you as soon as I found out.'

'Found out what?' I asked.

'Found out about the outcome of Karen's hearing. I couldn't call last night because it all finished so late. Plus I was out …'

'And the upshot?'

'Is that the kids are going back to her. She's been charged with wilful neglect, but they've agreed they can be returned to her, on condition that she accepts support from social services.'

So it was pretty much as anticipated. A formal rap on the knuckles, though she'd apparently argued her case pretty strongly, saying that in her opinion her daughter had been perfectly responsible and, aside from that ill-judged party, had cared for Jenson perfectly well.

But, in the light of so many recent and well-publicised incidents involving unsupervised children, the court had been firm. And I was glad of it. Compared to most of the families I had come into contact with professionally, hers wasn't that bad, but if what had happened could help in any way to repair the hidden fractures in their relationship, that had to be a good thing for all concerned.

'So when's it to happen?' I asked John.

'Pretty much ASAP,' he answered. 'Sunday was suggested –'

'*Tomorrow*?' It almost felt like a physical sensation.

'But I said no. I had a moment of complete inspiration. I figured Georgie into the equation and remembered what I'd been told about him. And my instinct was that it wouldn't give you enough time to prepare him for the upheaval. So I said Monday. No sooner. Did I do good, miss?'

I tried to laugh, but at the same time I felt sadness wash over me. Forget Georgie – it wasn't enough time to prepare *me*! I tried hard to swallow the lump in my throat so I could answer, and John must have sensed I wasn't dealing with it very well.

'It's okay, Casey,' he said into the silence. 'I know it's a shock. It always is when it's a case like this, isn't it? Though, thinking about it, also a bit different from your usual kids, I suppose. Arrived suddenly, gone equally suddenly. Which is unfortunately – or fortunately – something that happens from time to time. They turn up out of the blue, barely have a chance to unpack and then they're off again before you can say – oh, I don't know … "behaviour modification programme".'

That did raise a laugh. John had a gift for that, some-times. But only a small laugh. 'God,' I said. 'I am really going to miss him. Something I never thought I'd be saying a few weeks ago.'

'I know. It must be hard. Jenson's really settled in now, hasn't he? Look, I'll get off now and give you the chance to absorb all this and let everyone know. I know it's Sunday tomorrow but I've asked Marie to give you a call in the morning about everything. Ten okay? And could you give me a quick bell so I'm up to speed with the arrangements?'

I said yes, that was fine and that I would, and then good-bye, and then, still slightly stunned at the suddenness of everything, I fished around in the bottom of my bag for my fake cigarette. It was at times like this I was grateful I always carried it around with me, otherwise I'm sure I'd have gone straight to the nearest shop to buy some of the real ones. However intense the moment, I really didn't want that. *Get over yourself, Casey*, I told myself. *This is the way it works. They come, they go again.* Shouldn't I be getting used to it by now?

I could see Riley looking out for me from her table so I went back inside and told her the news. We both looked over at Jenson as I did so, at the natural and familiar way he now played with Levi, and I felt so sad that he had lost his little sister. He was such a good big brother; so gentle and attentive. And if I was seeing him through a filter of senti-mentality, then so be it. It was thinking this that I realised that it wasn't just that you never got used to a child going – there was an extra layer of feeling here. Shock, perhaps, because I never expected to feel like this? Plus was I compensating now for how poorly I understood him at the beginning? I didn't know. It was *always* tough when a child had to leave, but I honestly had thought that I hadn't been so attached to Jenson. After all it had only been weeks, rather than many months, that he'd been with us. Yet here I was, feeling bereft. Wrong again.

If I felt sorry for myself, I should perhaps have given more thought to how Georgie would cope with the news. When I sat down and told the pair of them, at teatime that same afternoon, the poor lad looked completely confused. I knew he was upset, but I hadn't figured on just how diffi-cult he'd find it to process it. We had no freak-outs; he was just so, well, troubled. While Jenson, naturally, was over-joyed to be seeing his mum again, Georgie spent the rest of the weekend wringing his hands together, walking around the house, head bent, with a painful expression on his face, muttering, 'Jenson going home. Jenson going away.' He also kept going upstairs without warning and spending minutes at a time just staring at Jenson's photograph on the bathroom door. And every time one of us approached him, he would just look at us in confusion. '*This* is where Jenson stays,' he kept repeating. 'That's his picture.'

I could have cried to see the state he was in, and, try as we might, we simply couldn't make him understand. By late Saturday night, when he couldn't settle down to sleep, I did wonder if I should ask for him to be put into respite for a couple of days to save him the anguish of the actual parting.

But when I phoned my Georgie lifeline, Sylvia, she asked me not to do this. 'This is real life, Casey,' she explained, with her usual wisdom. 'We never wanted Georgie to be institutionalised. I know he was living in one, so it might seem contradictory, but we always knew it wouldn't help him when the time came for him to leave us, so we tried to expose him to reality as much as we could. He needs to experience loss just as much as any other kid. I know you want to protect him from it, but it's inevitable, isn't it?'

She was right, of course, and, reassured now, I decided to stick with it. We'd just have to deal with the aftermath when it came about. Georgie *did* need to learn how to grow up as normally as possible – after all, he wouldn't be going back into a children's home when he left us. He'd be living with a normal foster family. Perhaps it was me who needed to man up – and let him take a few knocks along the way.

Marie phoned at ten on Sunday morning, as promised, and told me she would be driving Karen over to our house to pick Jenson up the next day.

'At around 11 a.m., if that's okay with you, so we can have them home by midday. Carley's foster parents are taking her home after lunch.'

I then phoned Riley and Kieron to invite them for Sunday lunch at our place so that the kids could spend a final day with Jenson. And it was a good plan: the afternoon was happy and uncomplicated, and the kids even bought Jenson leaving presents, bless them. From Riley and David there was another game for his beloved DS console, and from Kieron and Lauren a football shirt with his name emblazoned across the back.

He couldn't have been more excited. 'This is epic!' he exclaimed, with his usual understatement, before dashing upstairs to his bedroom and returning in full football regalia, complete with the floor-destroying studded boots.

But I didn't want to spoil the mood by carping on about it; my floors could cope with a few more scratches, I decided. Which was not the sort of thought I had that often, to be sure.

'Thanks, Kieron,' Jenson said shyly, once he'd finished hugging everyone. 'An' I was thinking. I don't live that far away, you know. So if it's okay with you I want to play in your junior team for real. You know, like *every* week. Properly, you're the best manager ever, an' I'll score loads of goals for us, I promise.'

I made another mental note to pass on this information to Karen's social worker. This was exactly the sort of parental commitment social services would be keen to promote. Kieron was busy wiping his eyes – the big softie. 'Course you can, mate,' he said, clearing the frog in his throat. 'You're already our lucky mascot. And if you keep it up you could become be our number one striker, as well!'

Even in the midst of this, Georgie seemed to be settling. Not wishing him to feel left out, Riley had bought him some *Doctor Who* figures, and he was engrossed within minutes of her giving them to him – setting a scene on the coffee table and speaking for each of his figures in turn, and even interacting in ways we had barely seen so far, chasing the little ones around the table with the silver Dalek figure and saying 'Exterminate' in his best scary voice.

We couldn't put off the inevitable, however, and, before I knew it, Monday morning was upon us. Jenson was quiet at breakfast, and when I went upstairs a bit later to help him finish packing, it was to find him staring out of his bedroom window. He turned as he heard me come in and I noticed he'd been crying.

'Saying goodbye's sad, isn't it, love?' I said, as I went and sat down on his bed. I patted the space beside me and he came and sat down himself, snuggling closer as I put my arm around him.

'It's like it's not real,' he said. 'It's like I've been here all this time and it feels like for ever. An' I'm going to miss it. I'm going to miss all of you.'

'We'll all miss you too, baby,' I said, struggling with my own composure now. 'More than anything. We've loved having you here. It's been *epic*.'

I sensed his smile. 'Casey, would you explain to Mum about me swimming? I want to keep going so bad, but not if it gets her all upset.'

'I promise,' I said. 'I'll tell her, love, and about your football too. I bet she's really proud of you. In fact, I know she is.'

He looked up at me. 'How d'you know that?'

'Because I'm a mum,' I said. 'And there are some things that mums know *all* mums think and feel. Trust me on that, okay?'

Which was a platitude, I knew, but an acceptable one, surely? 'Yeah,' he said, 'okay, but …' he faltered. 'You know Sammy?' Now it was me nodding. 'I couldn't help what happened to our Sammy, Casey,' he whispered. 'I *swear* it, I didn't know. I can't even really remember what happened. It's like it's gone …'

'You know, Jenson,' I said, squeezing his upper arm for emphasis, 'what happened that day – *whatever* happened – that day was *definitely* not your fault. You weren't much more than a baby yourself – you were only 5, love. And a lot of years have passed since then. These things take time, but I'm sure your mummy realises that it had *nothing* to do with you. And if she's grumpy, try to remember that she's not grumpy at you. It just hurts her to think about losing her baby, that's all. It's not *you*, I promise. Will you remember that?'

And all power to the social worker's elbow, I thought. Now they knew there was a problem, they could start to fix it.

By the time the car pulled up, Jenson was waiting at the front door with his new suitcase and proudly clutching his beloved 'stifficate' in his hand. 'They're here! They're here!' he whooped and shouted through the hall.

'Come on, sweetheart,' I said to Georgie, who was in the living room, studiously watching his beloved *Countdown*. That would be some challenge if they ever took it off air. 'Let's go say goodbye to Jenson, shall we?' I urged. 'He's going home now to be with his mummy. You remember me telling you about that happening, don't you?'

Mike had taken the morning off work and we could both see out of the window that he was now lugging Jenson's heavy case out to the gate. Georgie stood up and then made a sudden bolt for the stairs. *Oh well*, I thought, *I can't force him to face this if he doesn't want to*. I left him to it, and, plastering a polite smile on my face, went and joined Mike and Jenson in the front garden.

As people usually do, I had formed a mental picture of Karen but, as people usually find, seeing her in the flesh completely dispelled it. I don't think I'd been prepared for quite how much she looked like Jenson, or how young she seemed, or how vulnerable looking. But mostly how much her dead baby sprang to mind, and how my heart went its own way and went out to her.

She was very nervous, to the point that her hands were trembling as she shook ours. 'Thank you, *so* much,' she said shyly, '… for all you've done for him and everything. He thinks a lot about you, so … thanks.'

'You're welcome,' I said warmly, 'you really are. 'It's been a joy to have him. He's no angel, but he's a lovely little kid, he really is.' I grinned across at Jenson, over at the car, with Mike and Marie, busy loading it. I watched as he shoved the green holdall he'd come with into the luggage space above the back seats. Where had the time gone? It suddenly felt like yesterday. 'Look,' I added, 'I don't know if you knew, but when we took him to Wales on holiday Mike taught him how to swim. He's really good at it, too, and wants to know if he can keep it up.'

There. I'd said it. And it had struck a definite chord. That was clear. Karen looked directly at me. 'I suppose you know what happened to my little girl, don't you?' I nodded. 'So you can … well …' she shrugged. 'I'm sure you probably understand why I've never, well …'

'Of *course* I do,' I said quickly. 'Of *course* I do. But he *loves* it.' Now it was my turn to look at Karen pointedly. 'And it's done wonders for his confidence, and he really wants to keep it going. And maybe you could also … I don't know …'

'I know,' she said, nodding. 'And I'll try. Honest I will.'

Which had to be sufficient. It was work that could be continued by the social worker. Right now they had to head off. I could see Marie looking at her watch.

Jenson, however, was disappearing back into the house again. 'Jenson, love,' I called to him. It's time to get going …'

He turned. 'But where's Georgie? I have to say goodbye to Georgie.'

'Georgie is here,' said a voice from behind the front door.

'Come on then, you div!' Jenson laughed. ''Cos I'm heading off now. You gotta come out an wave an' that,' he said, pulling a reluctant Georgie out through the door.

'Present,' Georgie said, and at first I thought he meant *he* was present. But no, in his hand he had his own gift for Jenson. He opened his palm. It was a silver-grey, highly polished stone. 'A for ever stone for Georgie's for ever brother Jenson,' he said solemnly.

I could see Karen watching this exchange with some confusion. Which was a measure, I decided, of quite how far Jenson had come. This was now his normal, which could never, ever be a bad thing. Nor could what he did next, which was to fling his arms round a startled Georgie, and, while his for ever brother stiffened like a board, gave him a bear hug. And when he released him I thought I could see tears in Georgie's eyes.

'Thanks, bro,' he said, patting him. 'See you at school, mate, okay?'

And with that – and I could see that he didn't want to prolong the agony – Jenson ran to the car, jumped in and slammed the door.

The car had begun to disappear in seconds, leaving me with one clear impression to hang on to: of that luminous, bilious green holdall. I gulped a few times, and automatically put my arm around Georgie. But he was having none of it – he'd clearly had enough manhandling for one day. So while he went indoors Mike and I formed the small farewell party, waving and smiling as the car headed off down the road.

'I'm sorry, love,' I sniffled, 'I'm an emotional wreck, I really am. I don't know what's wrong with me today.'

'Well, you better brace yourself, love,' he said, as we followed Georgie inside. 'One down. Still another one to go.'

Chapter 22

However much, as a foster carer, you must expect the unexpected, sometimes you have to expect the expected as well. It was always the same when a foster child left the family. The house felt much too quiet, the vacated bedroom one room too many and the days seemed to drag like an old lady's bloomers. But it was to be expected. It was a period to be got through.

But, for some reason, particularly since he'd been with us a relatively short time, Jenson was proving to be a hard child to get over. Every now and then I would come across something that had belonged to him – an old sock at the bottom of the laundry basket, or his well-chewed school pencil – or I'd see his grinning photograph, which now adorned my living-room wall, smiling down among the photos of all the other kids. I would then have to force myself not to dissolve into tears. I was convinced I must be going through the menopause, I was that emotional.

But as Riley pointed out when I moaned on at her about it, Jenson wasn't like any of the other kids we'd looked after. He didn't come with half of the emotional baggage and we'd always known exactly where he'd be going back to. Therefore, Riley reasoned, we hadn't really seen him as a 'looked-after' child; we had taken him into our hearts and our family just as we would if it were a niece or a nephew, and this is what had made it all so difficult. I didn't know if I agreed with her or not, but it kind of made sense, so I went along with it. Better than the other explanation!

Georgie's reaction after Jenson left puzzled me as well. Despite the emotional display on the doorstep, ten minutes later, when we'd gone in and made a restorative cup of coffee, it was if he'd forgotten all about it.

'Here, Casey,' he'd said to me a couple of days later. 'Georgie good boy. Georgie helping doing housework.' I'd smiled as he'd handed me a crumpled mound of paper. I opened it up to find that it was actually two photos of Jenson, one from the bathroom door and the other from his bedroom.

'Oh, thanks, sweetheart,' I said. I didn't know what else to say really. 'But wouldn't you like to keep these in your special box?'

Georgie looked at me blankly. 'There are fixed points throughout time where things must stay exactly the way they are,' he said. 'This is not one of them. The eleventh Doctor.' He then dropped his head, clasped his hands behind his back and walked away, leaving me open-mouthed.

I stared after him. *Did this kid actually realise what he was saying? Did he try to select the correct quote to fit the occasion, or was it just luck?* Whatever the answer, that particular bit of mish-mash was uncannily apt.

Due to our impromptu holiday, I hadn't yet met up with Georgie's social worker, Mandy Heseltine. We'd spoken on the phone a couple of times and she seemed really nice and, most importantly, very enthusiastic about working with Georgie. So I was pleased to finally make an appointment to meet her and have the chance to put the face to the name.

It was the following Tuesday, just a week before school started – as if anyone who didn't know that could have missed it. The shops were no longer trying to offload all their summer-sale stuff, and instead were looking distinctly autumnal and back-to-work-ish – full of the usual reminders that it was time to knuckle down again: pencil cases, ring binders, racks of cardigans and jumpers, backpacks and lunchboxes and boots.

'Come in, come in,' I said to Mandy as I greeted her. 'I've explained what's happening to Georgie and he's waiting in the front room. I think he's a little nervous. He's been pacing.'

Mandy, who was very tall, very blonde and in her thirties, laughed as she followed me in. 'That makes two of us!' she confessed, and I immediately took to her. 'I was thinking – is it okay if I just say a quick hi to Georgie, and then you and I have a chat before I get to meet him properly?'

'Of course,' I said, understanding that a two-stage process might suit her better. Though we'd discussed Georgie on the phone, it still made sense to do it that way – she could grill me first and be better prepared.

I made a quick introduction and was as pleased as any mother that Georgie remembered his manners and held his hand out to shake. This was a recent accomplishment and a huge thing for Georgie. He found physical contact so difficult – and sometimes painful – but had been really trying to improve all his social skills so that he could be, at least superficially, a bit more like other kids. It was still all very stiff but, even so, a giant leap for him, and I felt a real sense of pride as I got him out some jigsaws before taking Mandy through into the dining room.

'Oh, wow – he's gorgeous!' Mandy remarked as we sat down with our coffee. 'He's on course to break a few hearts when he's older, for definite.' She sipped her coffee and grinned. 'But what about the maintenance? How on earth do you manage all that *hair*?'

'I actually haven't tried as yet,' I admitted. 'I've been too scared. He washes and brushes it himself and he's really very good at it, but I've never attempted to take him for a cut, because his last care-home manager said it might be a bit of a nightmare. They used to have to build him up to it for days in advance, but even then he got upset when he saw bits of his hair falling off.'

I also told her about the incident when we'd had to take him to casualty, and how they'd had to gather up the hair they'd had to remove to check his wound, so that he could take it home to keep in his special box.

'Doesn't surprise me in the least,' Mandy reassured me. 'I have another one just the same. One of my other long-term case kids – he's autistic too.'

'I didn't know that. But, of course, that's why they'd allocate you to Georgie. And you probably know so much more about it than I do. It's been a steep learning curve for me.'

'Oh, I know,' she said. 'Always is.' And the way she said it and smiled at me made me think that perhaps I was missing something. 'And that's exactly why,' she went on, 'they've given me Georgie. I've been Joshua's case worker for almost eight years now and he's quite high on the autism spectrum. He's verbal autistic – do you understand that?'

'I think so.'

'So you know that, like Georgie, he's acquired the ability for speech, although, as I'm sure you've realised, a lot of it's simply imitation and echolalia.'

I nodded, and wondered why she was going into all this. Was she perhaps preparing me for putting him on some sort of programme?

'Anyway, Joshua – that's his name – although pretty high on the spectrum, is relatively high functioning, compared to many. He's 18 now and has moved into a unit with three other young adults – all with special needs, and under the care of a support worker.'

I still didn't get why she was telling me all this. But then it hit me. Were they planning to move Georgie to some sort of similar but child-centred unit?

'I see,' I said, not really seeing at all.

Mandy beamed. 'It's been quite a transition, of course – him leaving his foster parents. Nine years he was with them, and they are missing him dreadfully. Wonderful couple. No children. Absolute superstars. But he's moved on, and is doing well, and that's what everyone's been working towards.'

I smiled back at her, my brain finally catching up at last. 'Oh, I *see*,' I said again. 'And you know, that's *so* good to know, because me and Mike were only saying the other day how worried we were for Georgie's future. I never realised that people like him could eventually move on as adults and have some degree of independence.'

Mandy leaned forward and poured herself another coffee from the jug. She was beaming again. That's when it hit me, like a lightning bolt. We weren't talking about Joshua here. We were talking about *Georgie*. And about a place that might be suitable for *him*.

'So this couple,' I said, wondering how I could be so slow on the uptake, 'they have a Joshua-shaped hole in their lives, which could perhaps be filled by Georgie?'

'Precisely,' said Mandy, reaching into her laptop bag and pulling out a file. She flipped it open and turned to face me. 'Helen and Mark,' she said, fanning out a sheaf of photos.

I looked at the pictures, one by one – such a happy group of images. Happy snaps of what was clearly a happy life. The three of them on a boat, the three of them laughing and eating ice creams, the three of them paddling in the sea, and many more. All depicting such love. I felt my eyes starting to prickle, and quickly blinked to stop the inevitable. *Riley's wrong*, I thought. *This just* has *to be hormonal!*

'Casey, Helen and Mark are such wonderful people. We think they'd be the perfect carers for Georgie. He's around the same age as Joshua was when he joined them, except Joshua had a lot more problems, and they worked miracles with him, they really did. They are devastated that he's left – devastated – even though this was always the ultimate goal. But when the time came – well, you of all people know how it feels, don't you? So, yes, they definitely have a Joshua-shaped hole in their lives. So. How about it? Is it time to meet young Georgie?'

I nodded again. I was beginning to feel like one of those nodding dogs that you see in the back of cars. I simply couldn't trust myself to speak. I'd been so sure I'd have Georgie for a good few months yet. Never dreamed I'd be losing him so quickly after Jenson. And just after I'd got myself so blooming organised and found *the* best website about autism.

And Mandy, in her wisdom, could see that. 'And here's the best news,' she said. 'They'd love to meet you. And for you to go and visit Georgie any time you'd like to. They realise how important attachments are, no matter how brief and tenuous …'

'What about school?' I asked suddenly, realising Georgie might be spirited many miles away. 'The attachment he has with Jenson, the other boy we fostered, is a really positive one. Incredible, really, given the short time they've been together. I couldn't bear it if he couldn't see Jenson again.'

Mandy's face fell. 'They live fifteen miles away, Casey. And there is a really good school near them. Joshua thrived there, honestly.'

Kick me, but I was beginning to get a little irked by this Joshua. This was about Georgie thriving. Georgie *and* Jenson thriving. *That* was what mattered to me. Mattered a lot. I decided to be assertive. 'If they understand about attachments,' I said, thinking on my feet and doing some mathematics, 'then they'll understand how important this particular friendship is. So my recommendation [*Hark at me*, I thought, *giving my professional opinion!*] is that, for the last year of primary school, transport is arranged so that Georgie is able to stay at his current school. It's not just about Jenson either,' I added. 'It's the whole sense of continuity he'll get from it. It's only one more school year – only nine months of minor inconvenience – and then he'd be moving up to secondary anyway. At least give him that time. It will be much better for him in a new environment. Particularly if he has Jenson as his constant.'

Mandy laughed. But in a good way. 'John Fulshaw said you might give me a hard time about this,' she said, grinning. 'Said you were a force to be reckoned with when it came to the kids.'

I felt myself blush. 'Oh, did he now?' But I was happy to laugh with her. Something told me that this might be a done deal.

'I will do my very best,' she promised me. 'In fact I really can see the benefit. Leave it with me.' She stood up then, towering over me. 'Right then,' she said. 'How about I go try to make Georgie understand our plan?'

The following Tuesday, the day before the autumn term started, we found ourselves once again on our doorstep, waiting for yet another social worker to tear our hearts out. I looked down at Georgie, who was looking down at the ground, hands behind his back, and reflected that this was something completely new.

Where he'd come to us with that singular 'cupping his hands in front of him' behaviour, that had been replaced with this new and different action. It made him look like a professor, trying to work out some important theorem, and it put me in mind of all the working out *we'd* had to do – and reminded that there was so much we still had to learn about him. The things he did, the ways he interacted, his very personality was so complex that you never knew, from one day to the next, what might be coming. But it wouldn't be us doing the learning now; it would be his new carers, and now he was going to them I really wished he wasn't.

Not yet anyway. Not that Georgie seemed that bothered either way, and seeing him smile, though I wasn't sure precisely what about, I was suddenly grateful for his lack of empathy.

Mike couldn't be with us today. An emergency at work meant he had to go in, and I felt, though we hadn't actually discussed it at all, that with Georgie it would be different – and perhaps not as traumatic, meaning he was safe to let me say goodbye alone.

Though not entirely alone. Kieron had come to see him off with me.

'You all right, mate?' he asked now, as he gently touched Georgie's shoulder. 'It looks like Mandy's here now. The car's arriving. See?'

I looked up to see it pulling up outside the gate. 'Kieron's right, Georgie, she is here. Are you happy?' Georgie just continued to smile, but at some point in the middle distance. 'You'll be seeing Jenson at school tomorrow, too.'

As I got no reaction to this either, I stopped talking. I'd won on that front, and I felt pretty chuffed to have done so. Georgie would be attending the same school for another year. Oh, but if only I could get one last tiny reaction …

'Mum, it's okay,' Kieron said, and he put an arm around my shoulder. For someone who was supposed to have problems with unspoken nuances, my son could read me like a book, he really could.

'Come on then, young man,' said Mandy briskly, as she came and joined us. 'Would you like to say goodbye to Casey and Kieron?'

She held her hand out, and, as if remembering a new important rule, Georgie took it, and then, also as if on cue – all my gentle training paying off? – he turned to us. I bent down. 'Is it okay if I give you a little kiss on your forehead, sweetie?' I asked him. 'I'm going to miss you but I'll visit you lots, I promise.'

Georgie smiled and nodded, and even let me kiss him without flinching. 'Time Lords, we have this little trick,' he then parroted. 'It's sort of a way of cheating death. Except

… it means I'm going to change. And I'm not going to see you again … Not like this. Not with this daft old face. And before I go … you were fantastic!'

And with that, he turned around and walked happily down the path with Mandy.

'Bloody hell, Mum,' gulped Kieron as we walked back inside. 'That's *harsh*.' He blew out a long breath, as if trying to dispel a bad sensation. 'I couldn't do that every few months. Are you okay?'

I nodded. 'Kieron, go and Google what Georgie just said, will you? I don't know how the hell he does that, but I'm sure it was *Doctor Who*.'

He did. And sure enough, it was exactly as I'd expected. 'Apparently,' Kieron read out loud, 'it was from the eleventh Doctor, and it was one of the most emotionally charged scenes of the series. The scene when he was saying goodbye to Rose Tyler.'

We were both momentarily speechless, trying to take it in, trying to absorb the meaning. And I think we might have succumbed to a bout of self-indulgent sentimentality, were it not for Kieron, who'd plainly had enough of that for one day.

'Lol!' he quipped, closing the lip of my laptop. 'Emotionally charged? They should try living in *this* family!'

Epilogue

Sadly, once home, Jenson's behaviour gradually deterio-rated. Though things started positively, and he continued to do well in primary school, his mother, Karen, never really co-operated with social services or came good on her promises to try harder with him.

The transition to high school the following autumn was a difficult one, and once there Jenson began truanting again regularly. He was placed back into care eighteen months later.

But perhaps this development, though we were obvi-ously sad to hear about it, was for the best. Much as we had hoped Karen might overcome her difficulties in relating to him, for Jenson it would only have been more psychologi-cally damaging to keep hoping for a love that wasn't there. He was placed with a lovely family in a different part of the country, and that's where he remains to this day. John updates us regularly on his progress and, the last time we heard, he was well and happy.

Georgie's local, of course, so we get to visit him all the time. Almost 12 now, he is such a lovely boy – still with his flowing locks! – and always seems to remember us when we see him. Never one to show much emotion, he still needs sensitive handling, but his foster mum tells us that whenever she tells him we are visiting he will pace the floor, hands gripped behind his back, like a little old man, just as he did the day he left us. She says he doesn't glance towards the window, but when he hears our car coming up the drive he sits down and smiles. That's good enough for us.

CASEY WATSON

*One woman determined to
make a difference.*

*Read Casey's poignant
memoirs and be inspired.*

Five-year-old Justin was desperate and helpless

Six years after being taken into care, Justin has had 20 failed placements. Casey and her family are his last hope.

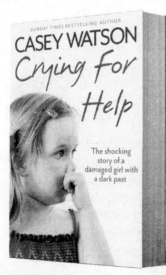

A damaged girl haunted by her past

Sophia pushes Casey to the limits, threatening the safety of the whole family. Can Casey make a difference in time?

Abused siblings who do not know what it means to be loved

With new-found security and trust, Casey helps Ashton and Olivia to rebuild their lives.

LITTLE PRISONERS

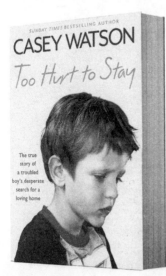

Branded 'vicious and evil', 8-year-old Spencer asks to be taken into care

Casey and her family are disgusted: kids aren't born evil. Despite the challenges Spencer brings, they are determined to help him find a loving home.

TOO HURT TO STAY

FEEL HEART.
FEEL HOPE.
READ CASEY.

Discover more about Casey Watson.
Visit www.caseywatson.co.uk

Find Casey Watson on **f** & **t**

WIN £500!

'Like' Casey Watson
on Facebook
for your chance to
WIN £500!

Simply find Casey Watson on Facebook
to enter into the prize draw and for full T&Cs.
PLUS get all the latest news about Casey
and her bestselling books!